Rise of the Patient Advocate

Healthcare in the Digital Age

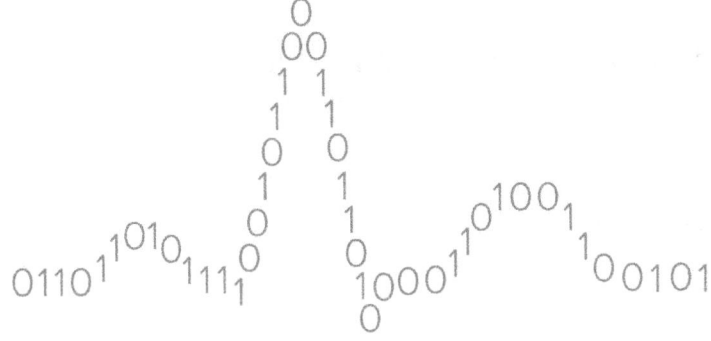

A guide to viewing and amending your electronic health record.

Showing you how to participate
in shared decision making that fosters
a strong patient-provider relationship.

Drs. Michael Warner & Margaret Warner

This book is intended to be an instructional guidebook for you, the patient. Names, characters, and medical scenarios are fictionalized for educational purposes. Any resemblances to actual individuals and/or medical events are entirely coincidental.

CONTENTS

Reviews

I have known Dr. Michael Warner for 20 years since his associate professorship at UMDNJ-SOM. He is a comprehensive family physician and patient advocate, utilizing the Osteopathic approach. Being the foremost critic in the field of EHR security and privacy in the age of the Internet, I believe that Dr. Warner is uniquely qualified to bring his experience to EHR to humanize and make relevant the use of medical data technology. "Big data" can be extremely positively powerful but it's misuse and disuse even more negatively powerful — even destructive. Drs. Warner are dedicated to making the use of healthcare data technology personal, relevant and safe, incorporating the elements of humanity.

Best wishes for good health,
Craig M. Wax, DO
Family physician, Editorial Board of Medical Economics
Host of Your Health Matters
Rowan Radio 89.7 WGLS FM

***

After 30+ years in healthcare administration, including physician practice management, hospital administration and BCBS payor management, I truly appreciate Drs. Michael and Margaret Warner providing not only the healthcare industry a guide to the future of medicine, but more important, giving the *consumer* (i.e., the patient/designated care-givers) a method of proactively managing his or her own healthcare through an on-line portal to better communicate health concerns and health status (too bad we had to wait for the government to legislate this kind of health promotion).

Dan Reaman, BSRT, MHA, NHA, Johnstown, PA

***

The Drs. Warner identify the revolutionary potential provided by the intersection of HIPAA, which provides patients with the right to access and amend their health records, with EHR portal systems, which provide the technical means for doing so on a large scale. They attempt to mold a movement through which patients improve their care by monitoring, correcting, and enriching their health records. It will be interesting to re-read *Rise of the Patient Advocate* in 30 years or so and bear witness to what extent the Warners' vision is realized.

Irv Freeman, Ph.D., J.D.
Vice President for LECOM at Seton Hill
Lake Erie College of Osteopathic Medicine

***

When I walked into my first medical school class, taught by Dr. Michael Warner, I knew I was in for an incredible experience. The medical education afforded to me in class took second rate to the lessons that Drs. Michael and Margaret Warner taught about patient advocacy and personal relationships in clinical rotations. After medical school, education from Drs. Warner continued and helped play a significant role in my becoming the osteopathic physician that I am today. Consequently, I cannot think of anyone more qualified to share their experiences and educate patients on participating in their own health records and health. *The Rise of the Patient Advocate* does a tremendous job in helping to bridge the gap between physicians and patients, which I certainly hope will improve an ailing medical system, in the midst of turmoil, for all patients and young physicians like me.

Kathryn G. Graham, D.O.
PGY-1 General Surgery, LECOM alumnus 2013
Arnot-Ogden Regional Medical Center, Elmira, NY

***

Drs. Margaret and Michael Warner's book *Rise of the Patient Advocate: Healthcare in the Digital Age* is an excellent, well-written guide that every patient and healthcare provider should read. In this age, when it is possible for healthcare facilities and independent doctors' offices to access the same health records, Drs. Warner show patients how they can be advocates for their healthcare through Electronic Health Records (EHR). The book covers many topics — from the benefits of EHR to the right to a universal pre-history to implementation of EHR. At each step, Drs. Warner show patients how they be active participants in their medical care. EHR's are becoming more commonly available to patients throughout our healthcare system. As they are implemented and used, this guide will be a great help to patients everywhere.

Pradip J. Shah and Ila P. Shah, Ebensburg, PA

***

In an era of evolving healthcare and physician constraints, it is time for patients to take on an active role in their own care. With access to their own records, it is both reasonable and plausible for patients to submit their own version of an outlined health history prior to their appointment. This would save the physician and staff valuable time, allotting more time to be spent on the more cerebral and personal aspects of medicine, for which the physician role is intended to be utilized, as well as affording patients more control over their care. It is a simple but powerful starting block for a more personal trend in patient advocacy.

Chad Metzger
3rd year Osteopathic medical student,
Philadelphia College of Osteopathic Medicine – Georgia Campus

I am looking forward to working in a healthcare environment that supports patient advocacy. I believe that the more input a doctor receives from a patient, the more efficient it will be to help diagnose and treat the patient. One of the goals I have while progressing through my education is to focus on learning and applying information and expertise to provide the best that I can for the patient. This is why I feel it is important to learn and understand as much as I can about patient advocacy in order to help realize this goal and eventually incorporate it into actual practice. As I enter my clinical years, I eagerly await being a part of the first generation of healthcare providers to encourage, support and practice patient advocacy.

Lara McGlynn
2nd year student Physician Assistant
St. Francis University, Loretto, PA

***

Acknowledgments

We thank our editor, Gabriella Gafni, J.D., for a wonderful experience. She became passionately attached to the revolution and helped us deliver our message.

We thank Mary Polito, C.R.N.P., D.N.P. for her heartfelt and enthusiastic participation in content and context!

Thanks also go to our family and friends who helped us develop this book to completion. We could not have done it without you.

We feel privileged to work with Mr. Scott Becker and Conemaugh-Duke Lifepoint Healthcare. Mr. Becker readily embraced this initiative as a means of improving the patient experience while empowering patient advocacy rights. We thank you for your leadership!

Our greatest thanks go to our patients. We have had the pleasure and honor of caring for people who have allowed us to be a partner in their healthcare experience. To you, we devote this book.

Foreword

Instantaneous medical information was once the material of science fiction novels and movies. Interplanetary doctors would wave wands over a suffering crew member and automatically deliver a diagnosis, treatment and cure. Meanwhile, in the real world, the health record lagged behind, as patient charts hung from clipboards at the bottom of hospital beds — a collection of notes and lab reports for the sole use of nurses and physicians. Entries were handwritten and filed in large folders and stored in a labyrinth of shelves. However, as we know, the only constant in this world seems to be change; and nowhere is this adage truer than in the world of healthcare. The advent of computers has made health records more current, thorough and easily accessed. The modern health record is no longer a sheaf of papers and reports. Rather, it is now a dynamic process that focuses on you, the patient, with the input of many professionals. Lab reports, treatment notes, and medications are still important entries, but now the patient has direct input and access to this most vital treatment tool. From almost any computer portal, patients are able to review, update, and comment on their treatment plans.

I invite you to learn more about how you can use this electronic tool to better serve you and more positively impact your medical care, treatment and hospital stay. Thanks to the hard work of Drs. Michael and Margaret Warner, you can take an active role in directing your own healthcare. The first step in this journey is just a page away.

Scott A. Becker, FACHE

Mr. Becker is the Chief Executive Officer of Conemaugh–Duke LifePoint Healthcare, Johnstown, PA.

Introduction

Like never before, you now have the ability to become more directly involved in the improvement of your healthcare. Newfound patient advocacy rights are emerging that allow you to control some of the content and most of the accuracy of your health record. This can be done through a patient portal connected to your doctor's Electronic Health Record (EHR) and with the use of a Universal Pre-History. In this guidebook, we will show you how to gain access to your health records, understand the content, and guard against inaccuracies. We will give you insight into electronic health record formatting to assist you in navigating the system and prepare you to be an active participant in your healthcare. We will explain how to review your records before and after every medical encounter and why this is important in your new role as your own patient advocate. We will also teach you how to get your story documented into the health record.

Healthcare in the United States is experiencing changes at many levels that are affecting all measurable parameters of quality, cost, and satisfaction. As family doctors and as patients, we have experienced these changes firsthand. We recognize that these changes are creating shifts in healthcare that will redefine typical approaches and long-standing expectations. We foresee the potential to improve national performance by having patients engage more significantly in their own care. One of the best ways to improve such care is for patients to communicate more effectively and efficiently with their healthcare providers. We believe that maximizing the use of your patient portal and "co-authoring" documentation in your doctor's electronic health record will accomplish these objectives.

The guidelines in this book will accomplish little if they are not applied. Doctors, nurses, receptionists, and everyone who has contact with patients has to follow a common set of rules when communicating – whether verbally, written, or electronically. We need to accurately capture and utilize pertinent health information for each patient. We have to function with consistency as both medical providers and patients contribute health information. For that reason, we have created this book as a reference and proposed guideline for everyone who contributes to the electronic health record.

As doctors, we want to understand our patients. This book highlights barriers and promotes solutions. As patients, we want to be heard. We want our information to be documented — sometimes in our own words — so as to best represent our needs.

Setting our approach apart from other recommendations and self-help aids, we offer solutions that will be scientifically tested. We are working with Conemaugh-Duke Lifepoint Healthcare in Johnstown, Pennsylvania to implement, study and research your new role as a member of the healthcare team.

You do not need to wait for our research to be done. The information in this book can readily be applied to the betterment of your health. We welcome the rise of the patient advocate, with you as an active participant in the healthcare experience.

Chapter 1

Why Should You Review Your Health Record?

Your Medical Story Is Important

Virtually everyone has a narrative — a unique story about their lives — thoughts, facts, emotions, predilections, ideologies, etc.; but few things are more important than the words written about you concerning your health. Shouldn't you be able to view, understand, and manage the information compiled in your health record?

Although computers have been in the financial and retail industries for decades, they are late to medicine. However, with modern, innovative technological advances such as electronic health records (EHR's), we are on the cutting edge of changing the ways in which doctors and patients interact with the personal information that literally lies at our fingertips. Even more significantly, understanding how to access and decipher your health records will enhance the doctor-patient relationship, while placing you and your doctor on equal footing when evaluating your medical needs and treatment options. This type of interaction will become a new standard in medical care, enabling you to become your own advocate. In so doing, you will empower yourself to make crucial decisions regarding your healthcare — and that of your loved ones — while fostering a meaningful dialogue with your doctor.

As a co-partner in the healthcare experience, you must be prepared to assess and control the content and accuracy of your health records, as well as correct errors and communicate your concerns to your doctor. This collaborative effort has the potential to bring forth higher satisfaction and quality, while lowering costs.

Because your health record is about you, no one understands your story better — even if some of the medical terminology may confuse or elude you. You should be able to speak to and inform your physician about inaccuracies in your health record, and participate in shared decision-making regarding your health.

It is our hope that as you read these pages, you will become the co-author of your personal healthcare narrative, able to create a roadmap to a healthier, more enlightened future.

Your Healthcare Wish Made Manifest: Doing Everything Possible to Improve or Save the Life of a Parent, a Child or Yourself

We are often presented with the question, "Why would patients be interested in reviewing their records?" The answer is simple: because they care about their health and the wellbeing of themselves and their loved ones; and, at the end of the day, they want to be able to say that they have done everything possible to improve or save the life of a parent, child, or themselves. Humans are forever hopeful and resilient — we strive to be invincible. One of the most important methods of "doing everything possible" now means reviewing your health records for content and accuracy. A mere office visit, which may last minutes, won't readily accomplish this objective. In fact, without the proper investigations and follow-ups with patients' health records, the precious resources of time and energy will be wasted — not to mention delays in treatment and the implementation of proper care.

Consider the following scenarios:

The Uninformed Patient

Cindy got a call from her doctor's office. The insurance company reviewed her health records and denied the MRI of her low back. This did not make sense. She has had terrible pains in her back and right leg for the past seven weeks. For the past month, her right foot has been weak, causing it to occasionally drag on the ground as she walks. She has attended physical therapy with little success and hoped to get a scan to discover the problem. Red flag: She did not know that her record lacked her complaints of pain radiating into her leg <u>with</u> foot weakness. She suffered with the pain for another month, and finally got the scan.

Had Cindy viewed her health records, she could have identified the missing pieces of information in her story. She could have brought this to the attention of her doctor. The documentation would have been accurate and her scan would have been approved the first time. She eventually needed a surgical procedure and has since recovered. Besides suffering with pain, she missed a lot of work, and almost lost her job.

***

Appearances Can Be Deceiving/The Importance of Medical Record Accuracy

Mary Ellen has multiple sclerosis. She used to play piano for every high school function, from choir to school plays. Over a period of three years, she had to drop back on her activities due to the worsening of her disease. When she dresses up, she looks great. Everyone who sees Mary Ellen remarks about her wonderful appearance. Little do they know that the two hours it takes for her to get dressed wipes her out for the rest of the day.

Mary Ellen collects social security disability. She reviewed her health records, which accurately describe her story. Despite "looking great," her records represent the actual severity and progression of her disease.

An accurate record is important for Mary Ellen. Beyond her healthcare, the record also maintains the status of her disability. If her record had read, "She looks great and is doing well," then her disability payments could have been terminated or, certainly, brought into question.

***

Speculation, Be Gone!

Patricia has been experiencing recurrent attacks of pancreatitis and has been hospitalized several times in the past year. She saw a specialist located three hours from her home. When she reviewed her health record, she did not find the consultation from the specialist. Upon calling the specialist's office, she discovered that her notes had been sent to her former doctor who is located in a town a hundred miles away! Fortunately, she was able to have the consultation letter sent to her current doctor.

Without the consultation letter in her chart, Patricia and her doctor would have wasted their follow-up encounter speculating as to the specialist's conclusions and recommendations. Result: a misuse of Patricia and her doctor's time, preventing timely access to the appropriate care.

***

The above stories speak to the issue of quality improvement, of which U.S. healthcare is in serious need. We would like to believe that our quality is the best, but our ranking indicates otherwise. On nearly every measurement scale of healthcare quality, U.S. ranking reveals a conspicuous lack of excellence. According to 2014 projections, the CIA World Factbook ranks us number 42 in life expectancy at birth when compared to two hundred twenty-three countries.[1] As to infant mortality rates (i.e., the number of deaths per one thousand births), the U.S. ranks 169.[2] The 2011 National Scorecard on U.S. Health System Performance by the Commonwealth Fund measured forty-two indicators and compared them with best practices internationally. Our country scored only 64 out of 100 points. This is a drop from 67 in 2006. The report explained that we needed a 40% improvement just to achieve benchmark levels of performance.[3]

---

1 The World Factbook. (2014, June 20). Retrieved November 14, 2014, from https://www.cia.gov/library/publications/the-world-factbook/rankorder/2102rank.html
2 The World Factbook. (2014, June 20). Retrieved November 14, 2014, from https://www.cia.gov/library/publications/the-world-factbook/rankorder/2091rank.html

The Commonwealth Fund's latest report, "Mirror, Mirror on the Wall – 2014 Update," ranked 11 countries for quality, access, efficiency and overall health. We did not score well. This prompted U.S. healthcare Forbes contributor Dan Munro to comment on the "Mirror, Mirror on the Wall Update" in his June 2014 article, entitled "U.S. Healthcare Ranked Dead Last Compared to 10 Other Countries."[4]

Public opinion polls show that Americans do not favor the quality of our healthcare system. A June 2014 Gallup Poll found only 44% of Americans rate our healthcare as either excellent or good.[5]

With regard to cost, our world ranking nears the top. With 2011 estimates, the CIA World Factbook ranks the U.S. #3 out of 190 countries for healthcare.6 The neighboring West African countries of Liberia and Sierra Leone take the number one and two spots. The Republic of Liberia (population: 4 million) consumed 19.5% of their Gross Domestic Product (GDP) to take the number one position, while the Republic of Sierra Leone (population: 6 million) took the number two spot with an 18.8% GDP. With the proliferating Ebola crisis, the percentage of GDP for Liberia and Sierra Leone will continue to rise. The United States used 17.9% of its GDP to take third place. When revising the list to include only large countries, the U.S. ranks number #1 in the world for cost. 2014 healthcare expenditures are around 18% of GDP, and are projected to reach 34% by 2040.[7] Financially, United States healthcare costs are on an unsustainable path.

3 Why Not the Best? Results from the National Scorecard on U.S. Health System Performance, 2011. (2011, October). Retrieved November 14, 2014, from http://www.commonwealthfund.org/publications/fund-reports/2011/oct/why-not-the-best-2011

4 Munro, D. (2014, June 16). U.S. Healthcare Ranked Dead Last Compared To 10 Other Countries. Retrieved November 19, 2014, from http://www.forbes.com/sites/danmunro/2014/06/16/u-s-healthcare-ranked-dead-last-compared-to-10-other-countries/

5 Newport, F. (2013, November 25). Americans' Views of Healthcare Quality, Cost, and Coverage. Retrieved November 19, 2014, from http://www.gallup.com/poll/165998/americans-views-healthcare-quality-cost-coverage.aspx

6 The World Factbook. (2014, June 20). Retrieved November 14, 2014, from https://www.cia.gov/library/publications/the-world-factbook/rankorder/2225rank.html

7 The Economic Case for Health Care Reform. (2014, June 9). Retrieved November 14, 2014, from http://www.whitehouse.gov/administration/eop/cea/TheEconomicCaseforHealthCareReform

Given our expenditures, we should, by all appearances, be satisfied with our healthcare. However, this is not the case. A June 2014 Gallup Poll showed that only 66% of Americans approve of the way the healthcare system works for them.[8] Interestingly, the poll's title is "Most Americans Remain Satisfied with Healthcare System." The term "most Americans" sounds good, but neither we nor our patients would be pleased with a 66% satisfaction rate in the medical office, the hospital or the emergency room. We believe that with the changing ways in which doctors and patients interact, these gloomy perspectives are about to change. The purpose of setting forth our knowledge and opinions, encapsulated in this book, is to promote your diligent review of your health record - before and after medical encounters - so as to check what is documented for content and accuracy. By doing so, you should gain a better understanding of what is happening to you and what to expect. To take your role as a patient advocate to the highest level, you require knowledge about how to craft and summarize your medical history, so that your doctor can be ready to do his or her part – for *you*. We show you how.

Being a co-equal participant in your care with your doctor signals a shift in your role, from passive to active. In order to address these new roles, we require new definitions of you, as a patient, and all of us, as our own patient advocates.

Let's examine the etymology of the words, "patient" and "advocate," so as to define the roles of each in the context of this presentation. The word "patient" derives from the Latin *patiens* (nominative masculine and feminine singular) and the Old French *pacient*, from the present participle of *patior* (i.e., "suffer," "experience," "wait"). As a noun, a *patient* is someone "who receives medical attention, care, or treatment."[9] Used as an

---

8 Newport, F. (2014, June 16). Most Americans Remain Satisfied With Healthcare System. Retrieved November 19, 2014, from http://www.gallup.com/poll/171680/americans-remain-satisfied-health-care-system.aspx
9 Patient. (n.d.). Retrieved November 20, 2014, from http://www.thefreedictionary.com/patient

adjective, *patient* means "to be able to accept or tolerate delays, problems, or suffering, without being annoyed or anxious."[10]

The word "patient" is shared in many languages throughout the world as a person who suffers with an illness or requires some kind of medical attention. In France, the term is used in the same context, but the "patient" is often referred to as a "client" (*client du doctor*).[11]

The word "advocate" stems from the Latin *ad* and *vocis*, meaning "from" and "voice." The standard definition of the word is "one that supports or promotes the interests of another." The Latin *advocatum* means "to call (oneself), to summon."[12] When the voice is heard, there is clarity. In the context of the doctor-patient relationship, we believe that the physician's objective is to listen to and hear the patient, and understand what he or she experiences by empathizing with the patient. We discuss the essential nature of empathy in Chapter 7.

"Patient advocacy" may imply "pleading for those who suffer;" but that definition characterizes the patient as weak. In our modern era, a new awareness should emerge that addresses the issues of illness and disease in conjunction with the right to be empathetically heard and understood as a client of healthcare.

As with every other service provider-client relationship — or in any sphere of life, for that matter — the foundation of a good relationship is based on mutual respect, trust, and the ability to cooperate. The partnership that you forge with your doctor is crucial, in that you and your physician are co-authors of the lifetime story of your health. Doctors want to hear your version of your narrative, and create a plan of action, tailored to your needs. This is not an ideal but, rather, an imminent reality, particularly when the patient is equipped with knowledge.

---

10 Patiens. (n.d.). Retrieved November 14, 2014, from http://en.wiktionary.org/wiki/patiens#Latin
11 Derived from a personal conversation with Jan F. Riguad, Ph.D., Retired Professor of French/Philosophy, Villanova University.
12 Jenney, Jr., C. (1970). *First Year Latin*. Boston: Allyn and Bacon.

Former Definitions:

Patient: "one who suffers and seeks medical attention"

Patient Advocacy: "pleading for those who suffer."

Modern Definitions:

Patient: "client of the healthcare system."

Patient Advocacy: "to exercise the right to be empathetically heard and understood while participating in shared decision-making that fosters a strong patient-provider relationship."

The Patient Advocacy Revolution: A Paradigm Shift

In "The Structure of Scientific Revolutions" (1962), American physicist, historian, and philosopher Thomas S. Kuhn, Ph.D. introduced the term "paradigm shift," signifying a change in basic assumptions — a revolution in thought and actions.[13]   Previous assumptions about your medical narrative are about to undergo enormous changes. Once off limits, your health records will be accessible, subject to your personal review, and manageable on your terms.

Embracing technology does not mean becoming ensnared in a web of bureaucracy.   Healthcare in the United States is in transition, and in the process, we must be ever mindful of three essential elements: quality, satisfaction, and cost. Together, you and your healthcare provider can create a clear record of your health that will promote your health and the good of countless others in the human family. When overall quality, satisfaction, and cost are at an optimum level, everyone will benefit. Your more interactive role as a patient will bring greater satisfaction and a higher quality of care. As this new approach evolves and becomes the standard, our healthcare system will become more cost-effective. As Dr. Kuhn noted, "A new way of looking at something becomes successful only when the old way miserably fails." Our healthcare system has failed

---

13 Kuhn, T. (1962). *The Structure of Scientific Revolutions*. Chicago: The University of Chicago Press.

in many ways, but is poised for dramatic improvement and redemption, with you at the helm, serving as a patient advocate for yourself and those you love. The time has come to view healthcare in a new way. Join us, as we traverse the path to better healthcare for all.

Chapter 2

Your Lifetime Health Story

What Is Your Health Record?

*Y*our health record is a lifetime story of your health. It is a living documentary of your life, in health and disease. Though this is a great definition, it is not in practice yet. Old concepts of the chart still prevail. The conversion to the new definition will occur as you become an active caretaker of your health record. As your own best patient advocate, it is up to you to keep it accurate.

At first glance, your healthcare decision-making rights may appear obvious, but the advancement of information technology has only now begun to empower us to exercise such rights. These rights are reaffirmed by the Privacy Rule, which became a final rule of HIPAA in 2002. The full name of the Privacy Rule is the Standards for Privacy of Individually Identifiable Health Information. The Privacy Rule clarified HIPAA's stance on our health care rights as patients, stating that everyone has the right to request to access our records and amend the content (45 C.F.R. § 164.524 access, 45 C.F.R. § 164.526 amend).

Many in the health care field remember when HIPAA was enacted. HIPAA, the Health Insurance Portability and Accountability Act of 1996, created an avalanche of regulatory paperwork to demonstrate that your health information was stored and transmitted securely.

With the Privacy Rule, HIPAA now extends beyond safeguarding your record as protected health information (PHI). It now calls for patient engagement and coordination of care with your medical provider.

The Advent of HIPAA

HIPAA empowers you with the right to obtain a copy of and request amendments to your health information, and protects your right to privacy.[14] We consider the law to be a reformation in patient advocacy.

Along with the prevalence of electronic health records (EHR's) came growing concerns about privacy, security, and storage. HIPAA directly addressed these issues.

Medical information can only be accessed by the patient, medical personnel, personal representative(s) and people processing your medical insurance claim.[15] Violations of Federal law involving improper viewing or alterations of your medical information carry stiff penalties. HIPAA, therefore, revolutionized the way in which the lifetime story of your health is reviewed, assessed, and managed. Your health record, therefore, is no longer limited to triggering your doctor's memory. Rather, the record prompts *you* to act, charging you with the task of active management of your healthcare narrative and, thereby, forging a more equal partnership with your doctor regarding your healthcare.

In the grander scheme of things, your health record now has a more far-reaching *public* impact than ever before. When aggregated with the general population, your health record creates information about health and disease, which is utilized by such agencies as the U.S. Centers for Disease Control and Prevention (CDC) and the World Health Organization (WHO). The results of data mining will provide a clear picture of where we stand regarding health and disease, while predicting future trends. In order to move forward with our sights on the future, it is important to

---

14 The HIPAA Privacy Rule and Electronic Health Information Exchange in a Networked Environment. (n.d.). Retrieved February 26, 2015, from http://www.hhs.gov/ocr/privacy/hipaa/understanding/special/healthit/correction.pdf

Your Health Information Privacy Rights (n.d.). Retrieved February 26, 2015, from http://www.hhs.gov/ocr/privacy/hipaa/understanding/consumers/consumer_rights.pdf
15 We will address the government's ability to view your information in Chapter 8.

look over our shoulders at how things were done and, subsequently, have changed.

Practices and Perceptions of the Past

At one time, health records were doctors' handwritten memory aids, sometimes in the form of three-by-five-inch cards, stored in a drawer. Documentation was simple and to the point. For example, "October 25, 1976 OM Amoxil" signified "The patient has an otitis media (OM) ear infection and amoxicillin antibiotic was prescribed."

Who would ever think that, one day, that little card would explode into an avalanche of paperwork? Due to subsequent mandates that supported billing, coding, and quality control, that is just what occurred. Charts became dense, voluminous stacks of information — often larger than big city phone books — piled throughout an office.

Human Curiosity

We should be curious about the content of our health records, as curiosity is an inherent human trait. It should be natural for us to want to see what has been written about us. Though we are accustomed to seeing laboratory orders and educational instructions, we have not routinely seen what the doctor has written about us. Now, you will be able to see every word concerning you, with only a few exceptions, which are detailed later in this book.

You should not be afraid or intimidated by your curiosity. In Latin, *cur* is the root for curiosity meaning "why?" We encourage you to be curious, so as to continuously seek answers.

The Purpose of Reviewing Your Health Records

Aside from being enshrined in the federal HIPAA law, there is a fundamental human right to know and access answers. After all, you are the focus of your health record, and since no one knows and understands your life story better than you, you have a right to ensure its accuracy. While it is true that you will not understand every aspect of your documents (e.g., blood tests and reports), you have comprehensive insight into your history, difficulties and health concerns. If you had a hysterectomy, for example, surely, you would be familiar with the term; and if you had a meniscal knee tear, you would most likely know a great deal about that, as well. In this age of advanced information technology, *everyone* (including patients) has a heightened awareness of a vast array of subjects. Your medical information is one of the most important – if not the *most* significant — source of knowledge that you can access.

EHR's: *Mandatory Use, Access, Incentives and Penalties*

We believe that since your lifetime health story is essential to the continuance of your care and treatment, reviewing your record will, in the near future, not only be voluntary, but *mandatory*, as is the digitalization of health records. In 2012, only 17% of U.S. physicians were using advanced EHR systems, as compared to 78% in 2014.[16] Over the past several years, the government and insurance companies have offered financial rewards to healthcare providers who adopted and used EHR's. Beginning January 1, 2015, doctors not using the new system experience financial penalties under certain federal healthcare programs.

In 2013, physicians had an opportunity to earn an extra 0.5 % bonus for their offices, if quality measures were completed. This amounted to a fifty-cent incentive payment for every one hundred dollars earned by a medical practice. Since the beginning of 2014, doctors received 2.0% penalties if quality measures were not completed. Though reasonable, the lists, as applied, are sometimes unsound. At times, insurance companies creatively promote physicians incentives with some rules that are nearly impossible to achieve.

---

16 Doctors and Hospitals' Use of Health IT More than Doubles since 2012. (2013, May 22). Retrieved November 14, 2014, from http://www.hhs.gov/news/press/2013pres/05/20130522a.html

Identifying and Implementing Quality Measures

Mechanisms are in place to promote fairness, compensation, and partnership in health with your doctor. If you receive a flu shot outside of the doctor's office (e.g., at a pharmacy or at work), your healthcare provider should use this code: *G8482 influenza vaccination given elsewhere.*[17] This sends a message to the insurance companies and our government that you received your flu shot this season.

Some codes also exist to account for legitimate reasons why a quality measure cannot be performed. Such codes include: *Influenza vaccination withheld due to allergy (v64.04)* or *patient refuses immunization (v64.06).*[18]

Incomplete Quality Measures and Patient Penalties

You should work with your doctor to complete all required quality measures. If not, penalties soon may apply to *you*. We already witness insurance companies' increasing cost for higher premiums and co-pays when quality measures are not completed. In the near future, you may have to ensure completion just to keep your insurance.

Some employers now require all employees to get a yearly flu shot in order to remain employed. Legitimate excuses are accepted, but they must pass a review board. You cannot go to your doctor, present a vague excuse, and receive a waiver.

While employer mandates can easily provoke debate, we see little conflict over quality mandates from the medical side. Patients with hypertension must have their blood pressures monitored. Their cholesterol and kidney function should also be tested at least once a year. As a co-partner in health, ask your doctor to list all of the required measures

---

17 *2014 HCPCS Level II Expert.* (2013). American Association of Professional Coders (AAPC) Edition of the Centers for Medicare & Medicaid Services Healthcare Common Procedure Coding System (HCPCS) Code Set.

18 *2014 ICD~9~CM Expert for Hospitals & Payers* (AAPC Legacy Edition of the International Classification of Diseases, Ninth Revision, Clinical Modifications ed., Vol. 1 through 3). (2013). OptumInsight.

for your individual healthcare needs. Complete the measures, and be sure that they are documented in your health record.

Your Communications Become a Permanent Part of Your Record

In the digital age, through online portals, you can now perform such activities as scheduling appointments, requesting medication refills, or asking a question. In the latter instance, however, you have to ensure that, when posing a query, you express your exact intention. What you write becomes a permanent part of the record, and will be forwarded to a staff member who, in turn, will present it to the physician (if need be).

Your health record not only shines a light on your past and present health history — labs, treatments, and general condition but, also, your refusal or consent to receive certain types of treatment. Remember that you now have the right to be the co-author of your health destiny, and your intentions must be expressed.

The Implications of Refusing Treatment

The right to refuse care should be universally acknowledged. You can refuse *any* form of treatment (e.g., chemotherapy, dialysis, etc.) — as long as the refusal does not affect or endanger anyone else. A person who has contracted the Ebola virus, for example, cannot refuse quarantine, due to the dangers that a lack of isolation can pose to others. Refusing the flu shot can be a sticking point. If you are over age sixty-five, if you have diabetes or asthma, getting a flu vaccination becomes imperative. Not getting the immunization puts you and others at physical and also financial risk, given the costs associated with taking care of influenza patients. When compared to hospitalization or an emergency room visit, a flu shot is inexpensive. If you opt not to be immunized and you contract the flu, you could become ill and spread the virus to others. Every year, about twenty-five thousand Americans die from influenza.[19] Companies are concerned about costs associated with lost days of work due to the illness and higher costs associated with taking care of a sick person. Curiously, you have a right to refuse influenza vaccination, but in some places of employment, you do not have a right to work if you refuse the shot. We anticipate that future insurance models will begin to discount co-pays and premiums for all customers who opt for the yearly vaccination. This will, in turn, escalate costs for those who refuse it.

Most medical decisions involve greater difficulties than whether or not to get an influenza vaccination. For example, what are the benefits of certain medication or surgery? What are the risks? and, of most importance, the question asked, in a face-to-face discussion, "If I choose this option, what will happen to me?"

A corollary of your right to accept and refuse certain types of treatment is your decision-making power, enshrined in an advanced healthcare directive. This determines the nature of your *future* care — particularly focused on when you are not be able to speak for yourself. Such is one of the rights conferred by The Patient Self-Determination Act (PSDA, 1990).[20]

The PSDA Confers the Following Rights:
The right to facilitate your care
The right to accept or refuse medical treatment
The right to make an advanced directive

---

19 "Estimates of Deaths Associated with Seasonal Influenza – United States, 1976-2007, Morbidity and Mortality Weekly Report (MMWR), Centers for Disease Control and Prevention (CDC)", August 27, 2010, vol 59, 1057-1062.
Influenza viral infections kill about 23,607 Americans every year. The number has varied from 3,349 in the 1986-1987 flu season to 48,614 in 2003-2004.
http://www.cdc.gov/mmwr/preview/mmwrhtml/mm5933a1.htm

20 Patient Self-Determination Act. (n.d.). Retrieved February 26, 2015, from http://en.wikipedia.org/wiki/Patient_Self-Determination_Act

Formerly the Omnibus Budget Reconciliation Act of 1990, this law applies to all States, and requires that an advanced healthcare directive be given to any person upon admission to a healthcare facility. The PSDA does *not* apply to sole practitioners or to those who work in an independent group (not owned by the hospital or a health system).

Under the PSDA, a patient has the right to facilitate his or her own healthcare decisions, to accept or refuse medical treatment, and to make an advanced directive. An advanced directive allows someone to document specific healthcare instructions in the event that they may not be able to communicate. These instructions can describe how you would want to be treated. Would you want to have Cardiopulmonary Resuscitation (CPR)? Would you want to be on a ventilator? Would you want certain music to be played and never "certain" other types of music? These are important issues and you should think about them every so often.

You also need to think about your surrogate(s). If you are lucky enough to have someone who cares about you, then perhaps they should have some say as to how you are treated. Being a surrogate can be stressful, but it is always honorable. To take some stress off of your surrogate, keep your health records organized and up to date. Your surrogate will have difficulty helping you if your medical information is disorganized.Not all surrogates are able to follow and maintain your wishes. Sometimes, they cannot say "goodbye" and they cannot say "no." Therefore, make sure that your surrogate understands how you feel, and promises to carry out your intentions.

According to Daniel Wehner, M.D., M.B.A., Chair of Emergency Medicine, Conemaugh-Duke Lifepoint Healthcare, Johnstown, PA, "Advanced Directives, Living Wills and Durable Healthcare Powers of Attorney all have limitations, especially in the Emergency Department, where decisions and actions must be made quickly."[21] He adds, "If the information is not clearly stated, all healthcare professionals – from the

---

21 Schmidt, T. "Moral Moments at the End of Life," Emergency Medicine Clinics of North America, vol. 24, 2006, p. 787-808.

EMS team to the ER – are going to apply all means of resuscitation." Though federal law (PSDA) supports a variance of forms, Dr. Wehner recommends the use of a POLST for patients with terminal illness or severe chronic disease.[22]

The Physician Orders for Life-Sustaining Treatment (POLST) originated in 1991, when a task force of Oregon health providers and organizations sought "to develop methods for honoring patient treatment choices near the end of life." The POLST form is a *physician/provider order.* The document is divided into five sections. To complete, check one box for each of the first four sections. The form must remain with the patient when the patient is transferred to a different department within a healthcare facility or upon discharge. Because a POLST is an order and it accompanies the person, it is followed with the strictest of duty.

Physician Orders for Life-Sustaining Treatment (POLST)

Cardiopulmonary Resuscitation (CPR): Person has no pulse and is not breathing.
☐ Resuscitate/CPR
☐ Do Not Attempt Resuscitation (DNR/no CPR)
Medical Interventions: Person has pulse and/or is breathing
☐ **Comfort Measures Only** – use medication by any route, positioning, wound care and other measures to relieve pain and suffering. Use oxygen, suction and manual treatment of airway obstruction as needed for comfort. Do not transfer to hospital for life-sustaining treatment, Transfer if comfort needs cannot be met in current location.
☐ **Limited Additional Interventions** – includes care described above. Use medical treatment, IV fluid and cardiac monitor as indicated. Do not use intubation, advanced airway intervention, or mechanical ventilation. Transfer to hospital if indicated. Avoid intensive care.

---

22 Pirinea, H., Wehner, D., Simunich, T. , "Patient and Health Care Provider Interpretation of DNR and DNI," Conemaugh-Duke Lifepoint Healthcare, Johnstown, PA, not yet published.

☐ **Full Treatment** – includes care described above. Use intubation, advanced airway interventions, mechanical ventilation, and cardioversion as indicated. Transfer to hospital if indicated. Includes intensive care.

Additional orders: _____

Antibiotics

☐ No antibiotics. Use other measures to relieve symptoms.

☐ Determine use or limitation of antibiotics when infection occurs.

☐ Use antibiotics if life can be prolonged.

Additional orders: _____

Artificial Administered Nutrition: Always offer food by mouth if feasible.

☐ No artificial nutrition by tube.

☐ Defined trial period of artificial nutrition by tube.

☐ Long-term artificial nutrition by tube.

Additional orders: _____

Summary of Medical Condition and Signatures

Discussed with (check all that apply)

☐ Patient

☐ Parent of Minor

☐ Healthcare Representative

☐ Court-Appointed Guardian

☐ Other:

Summary of Medical Condition:

Print Physician/Nurse Practitioner Name:

Physician/NP Signature (mandatory):

MD/DO/NP Phone Number:

Date:

SEND FORM WITH PERSON WHENEVER TRANSFERRED OR DISCHARGED

Unlike the Advanced Directive, which is meant for anyone 18 years and older, the POLST is for persons with serious illness – at any age.[23]

These issues can, potentially, be intense and immediate — an explosive combination of events and emotions. Without hesitation, the entire healthcare system is there to support you and your wishes. The POLST form and how it is handled is an example of how we can use the current system to make things work.

Now that we have identified the nature of your healthcare narrative and your control over it, we will explore more ways in which the digital age is revolutionizing healthcare.

---

23 Lofgren, J., Catenacci, M., Bookman, K., "End-of-Life and Futile Medical Care in the Emergency Department," Emergency Medicine Reports, vol 35, No 22, October 19, 2014

Chapter 3

Healthcare In the Information Age

*M*uch of the information contained in this chapter is technical, but not beyond the reach of general understanding. We believe that it is vitally important for you, the patient advocate, to understand the nature of how data is being transmitted to and received by your doctor, so as to facilitate a more comprehensive, informed healthcare dialogue.

As data is becoming increasingly digitalized and consolidated, the amount and quality of information is expanding and changing. In this state of constant flux, an educated patient has a better chance to be a healthy patient. With this understanding, let's take a look at some important terms and practices.

Remote Patient Monitoring, Big Data and Quantified Self

The innovations are rife. Sleep apnea machines provide remote patient monitoring, as they can now send reports to the physician. Pacemaker recipients can send information to their cardiologists by holding a telephone next to their chests. Patients suffering from heart failure or obesity can monitor activity levels with wearable devices and can share information with their medical providers. With these technological advances, your healthcare record will, most likely, expand to include information regarding your actual diet, activity and mood. Therefore, you should be familiar with the latest terminology rapidly working its way into our everyday vernacular.

"Quantified self" involves tracking and analysis of every one of an individual's efforts in furtherance of self-improvement.[24] Ginger.io and Fitbit® are examples of "quantified self" tools. The former application requires physician approval and employs a smartphone application that actively and passively tracks and analyzes your existence. Passive data is collected by silently tracking what you do. Traveling, texting, web surfing and telephone call habits have been shown to vary on the basis of one's health status. People who feel good, interact with other people and move around in the world. Active data is amassed through short daily surveys, tailored to the individual's specific healthcare issues. Questions may include the following: "How do you feel today?" or, for patients with diabetes, "What was your fasting blood sugar reading?"

Ginger.io results have demonstrated a surprising near-identical overlap between passive data (i.e., what you did today) and active data (i.e., how you responded to questions about your health). Quite astonishingly, the system can detect a change in health more quickly with passive data than the active data. This means that the system's tracking of your voice calls, texts, and web surfing can signal a marked change in your health even before you would recognize or acknowledge it. Very soon, you will not have to wonder whether your elderly father has a change in his health status. Rather, you will receive a message, stating that he may not feel well, since he has not called anyone today, he has not changed the television station (there is no activity on the television's remote application), and he has not followed his grandchildren on Facebook. This will prompt you to call and ask, "Dad, are your ok?"

Fitbit® is one of numerous wearable products designed to track your activity. Fitbit Flex™ and Charge™, for example, are wristband devices that can measure activity and sleep patterns. By using Fitbit® tools, participants can make activity goals, as well as log caloric intake. Customers can even choose to compete with each other. Sensoria Fitness

24 Data Overload: Is the 'Quantified Self' Really the Future? (2014, August 30). Retrieved November 14, 2014, from http://www.nbcnews.com/tech/innovation/data-overload-quantified-self-really-future-n189596

has smart garments, ranging from t-shirts to sport bras and socks. The fabric of t-shirts and sport bras is embedded with sensors to measure your heart rate. Linked to a Sensoria® application on your smartphone, you can track the effectiveness of your workout. The socks are also embedded with sensors which precisely track activity, measure cadence, detect foot landing technique, and pick up center-of-balance information to improve your running form.[25]

"Big data" is a term used to describe the volume and complexity of health information generated by the digital age, which will allow for high-level analysis. The results of data mining will provide a clear picture of the state of health and disease, along with the prediction of future trends.

Present-Day Data Collection Problems

Although we want and have to monitor as much data as possible, our healthcare system has been measuring very little. Most of the data regarding the treatment of disease has come from "billing claims analysis." For decades, doctors have used the Health Care Finance Administration's HCFA 1500 form to submit medical bills (whether paper or electronic) to and through a clearinghouse vendor. Until recently, Field 21 in the 1500 form limited the amount of diagnostic codes to a maximum of four. This means that no matter how many problems you addressed at your medical encounter, your doctor has been limited to listing only four. There is a way to create an additional claim, so to gain another four slots. In coding lingo, it is called "dropping another claim." This is time-consuming and almost always denied. We view claims-based data as being incomplete and deceptive. Because of the four-problem limit, information derived from "claims data" should not be regarded as accurate or conclusive.

---

25 Smart Socks, Powerful Electronics. (n.d.). Retrieved November 14, 2014, from http://www.sensori-afitness.com

The National Uniform Claim Committee (NUCC) is an advisor to the Centers for Medicare & Medicaid Services (CMS), whose task (among others) is to implement updates and changes to the 1500 claim form. As of April 1, 2014, the NUCC recommended an expansion of the clearing house vendor limit of the 1500 Health Insurance Claim for processing field 21 from four to eight slots. This was done to increase the quality of claims-based data. When a 1500 form is submitted, it goes to the insurance company or the government though a clearinghouse vendor. Because NUCC is not a regulatory agency, some vendors dismiss an obligation to recognize more than four diagnostic codes. Beyond defying the recommendation of the NUCC, they claim that technical costs will be incurred if they re-program their system from four to eight slots. Can you imagine a department store warehouse limiting the amount of inventory that can be counted? In the medical field, we have a clear case for more information, but all of us are not on the same team. Without expansion beyond four codes, we cannot properly manage our healthcare system. To compound this existing problem, the data that is available to us is misleading.

Case study — Limiting Codes Stymies and Discredits Physicians, Narrows and Contaminates Healthcare Data

Dr. Henry sees his patient, whom he diagnoses with Diabetes mellitus, hypertension, high cholesterol, and migraine headaches. The patient has also developed a urinary tract infection. The latter diagnosis is corroborated by the symptom of urinary frequency and a subsequent urinalysis at the doctor's office.

In order to be paid for the urinalysis, the urinary tract infection code (599.0) must be submitted as one of the four top codes. In submitting the claim form, Doctor Henry has to be selective. He chooses diabetes (250.00), hypertension (401.1), migraine headache (346.90) and urinary tract infection (599.0) as the top four. Since the slots are limited, Dr. Henry is constrained not to submit high cholesterol (272.0). According to claims data reports, Dr. Henry does not care about cholesterol when treating patients with diabetes and hypertension.

During the office visit, the patient-doctor exchange is often very comprehensive, but the resultant data has artificially reduced that conversation to merely four codes of the billing form. Such narrowed, contaminated data has effectively stymied and discredited medical providers.

The Futility of Limiting Data

Limiting diagnosis data to only four slots makes our care look incomplete and renders claims data nearly useless. If a patient requires a strep throat test or a urinalysis, one or two diagnostic slots would be taken on the billing form. Pharyngitis (462) would be required to support the strep test, and urinary tract infection (599.0) or urinary frequency (788.41) would be required to support the urinalysis. If a patient refuses an influenza vaccination (v64.04), yet another slot is taken. To make matters worse, insurance plans want the Body Mass Index (v85._ _) to be submitted with each visit, so there goes another slot.

Increased Efficiency and Evidence Based Medicine

Data incompleteness and misrepresentation cost money, time, and lives. Consider, for example, the prevalence of Diabetes mellitus in our country. Unfortunately, claims data provides a skewed view of the disease, because of the limitations of Box 21. Diabetes is not always included in one of the four slots, even if it is addressed at the medical encounter. To make matters even more complicated, some diabetic codes require "linked codes" to be used. A patient with *controlled type II Diabetes mellitus with diabetic-related kidney and nerve disease* would require submission of four codes: 250.40, 585.3, 250.60, 337.1 — *exactly in that order.* If 250.40 were used alone, without being followed by 585.3, billing computer programs would reject the claim, and return it to the doctor, unpaid. Even if the doctor recorded the codes correctly, what are the chances that all four codes would be used in the four Box 21 slots, and what about the patient's other conditions?

Right now, when it comes to healthcare data in the United States, we are unequipped to know the extent of our resources. Consider an analogy to a stock room clerk at a large grocery store. The clerk can tell you exactly how many bottles of water are on the shelves and stored in the back. Unfettered by the number of computer fields in which the bottles can fit, the clerk inherently knows the extent of the store's inventory. The medical informatics clerk (doctor), however, is only allowed to count to four.

No wonder our healthcare system is in trouble! Without enough of the right data – and, worse, yet, too much of the *wrong* data — the system has become unmanageable.

With regard to effectively tracking health and disease in this country, the current system is lagging behind. Our system concludes that Dr. Henry (in our previous example) does not care about cholesterol when treating patients with diabetes and hypertension, but that is untrue. Experts could argue that American medical providers do not care about such conditions as renal (kidney), ophthalmic (eye), neurologic or circulatory manifestations when taking care of people with Diabetes mellitus. "Claims data" could conclude that doctors are incomplete and uncaring when taking care of patients with chronic diseases.

We caution any quick conclusions, until we obtain better evidence of what is wrong. Someone could easily conclude that our system would be better if we got rid of our fictional Dr. Henry, when in fact, we need more providers like him.

The term "evidence-based medicine" (EBM) was coined in 1987 by David M. Eddy, M.D., Ph.D.[26], to describe the research and analysis of information that allows medical providers to make wise decisions. In the

---

26 David M. Eddy, M.D., Ph.D. received a B.A. in History from Stanford University, Doctor of Medicine from the University of Virginia in 1968, and a Ph.D. in Engineering-Economic Systems from Stanford University in 1978. He has served as the Chief of the Bioengineering Branch of the U.S. Army Research and Development Command, Professor of Engineering Economic Systems at Stanford University, Professor of Health Policy and Management and J. Alexander McMahon Professor of Health Policy and Management at Duke University.

1970's, Dr. Eddy, also a mathematician, applied mathematical models to define criteria for cancer screening, which has led to the formulation of clinical practice guidelines for nearly every disease and condition.

We salute Dr. Eddy, while realizing that the greatest impact of his work will soon be realized. We will expand billing information so not to restrict input data. We will be able to use the entire digitalized electronic health record as an information resource.

United States Preventative Services Task Force (USPSTF)

Medical providers are continually educated in reference to evidence-based medicine (EBM). We recommend that you look to the United States Preventative Services Task Force (USPSTF) as a source of evidence-based medicine guidelines. USPSTF is comprised of a panel of physicians and epidemiologists (i.e., scientists who study the patterns, causes, and effects of health and disease in a defined population) appointed by the United States Department of Health and Human Services' Agency for Healthcare Research and Quality.

Doctors use USPSTF for recommendations as to when and whether to order preventative tests, such as mammograms or prostatic specific antigen (PSA) blood tests. You can view current and upcoming recommendations via this URL: http://www.uspreventiveservicestaskforce.org.

The good news is that as information is less restricted, crippling medical data will be replaced with valuable information. Just as in other industries, healthcare will be positively impacted by the information revolution; and when you combine that flow of information with your ability to review and amend your record, we witness an enormous paradigm shift.

Why Pessimism Prevails Among Doctors

Although trends look promising for medical data, doctors are pessimistic about the future of medicine. Over 84% of physicians agree that the medical profession is in decline.[27] This statistic reflects the opinions of over eight hundred fifty thousand physicians (M.D. and D.O., alike)[28] in the United States. This near-million number does not include physicians' assistants (P.A.), certified registered nurse practitioners (C.R.N.P.), Certified Registered Nurse Anesthetists (C.R.N.A.), Professional Midwives (C.M., C.N.M., C.P.M., D.E.M.)[29], Doctors of Nursing Practice (D.N.P.), Doctors of Optometry (O.D.), Doctors of Chiropractic Medicine (D.C.) and Naturopathic Doctors (N.D.) who might step forward in agreement. This level of despair ensues from the fact that medical providers face a system that punishes them for doing more for their patients, and undermines comprehensive care. Consequently, they feel disconnected from their mission to help patients achieve their optimum health.

Case Study — Bundled Payments

Joe saw his doctor for a chronic disease encounter. His hypertension is controlled with medication, diet and exercise. His blood pressure and routine blood tests results are good, and a medication refill was ordered. A couple of years ago, his prostatic specific antigen (PSA) was mildly elevated. During the present visit, Joe and his doctor discuss the risks and benefits of further prostate testing, and Joe concludes that he wants to live the rest of his life without worrying about it. While speaking with his doctor, Joe also complains of right knee pain and arthritis, which causes difficulty in walking. His doctor gives a steroid injection into his knee during the visit. Joe reports feeling better that day, and by the weekend,

---

27 Hawkins, M. (2012, September). A Survey of America's Physicians: Practice Patterns and Perspectives. Retrieved November 14, 2014, from http://www.physiciansfoundation.org/uploads/default/Physicians_Foundation_2012_Biennial_Survey.pdf
28 Medical Doctor or Doctor of Medicine (M.D.), Doctor of Osteopathy or Doctor of Osteopathic Medicine (D.O.)
29 Certified Midwife (C.M.), Certified Nurse-Midwife (C.N.M.), Certified Professional Nurse Midwife (C.P.M.), Direct-Entry Midwife (D.E.M.).

he feels "great." Joe's insurance company paid the doctor for the injection, but not for the office visit.

The government and insurance companies are concerned that doctors will perform too many procedures; so, when many issues are addressed all at once, they often "bundle" the payments.

The Current Procedural Terminology (CPT®) manual is the physicians' procedural rulebook.[30] The manual instructs physicians to add CPT Modifier 25 to the 1500 Claim to recognize a "significant, separately identifiable evaluation and management [E/M] service by the same physician on the same day of the procedure or other service." This allows the provider to both perform a procedure and conduct an office visit. Very often, however, the government and insurance companies elect to ignore the modifier and pay only for one service per day.

Case Study — Patient Inconvenience, Curtailed Care

Edward visits his doctor for chronic disease management of his atrial fibrillation and hypertension. He takes Coumadin daily to reduce the risks of blood clots and strokes. During the examination, the doctor discovers impacted ear wax in both ears. Edward attributed his hearing loss to hearing aid malfunction. The doctor contemplates immediate removal of the ear wax, but decides to send Edward to a specialist. Ear wax removal is time-consuming and, in the past, the doctor often did not get paid for the procedure.

The problem lies in the fact that Edward's insurance company does not want to pay an extra thirty dollars to the family physician for ear wax removal while he is at the office for disease care. The insurance company will, however, pay multiple times the amount for the patient to see a specialist. This is an inconvenience for patients who, like Edward, must

---

30 *Current Procedural Terminology CPT®* (2014 Professional Edition ed.). (2013). American Medical Association.

see another doctor and remit another co-pay. Although this fact does not sound logical, the insurance company reaps the benefit. Because most family doctors want Edward to hear right now, they will remove the ear wax whether they receive compensation or not — hence saving money for the insurance company, which avoids payment for the service altogether.

This should not evoke discontent between primary care physicians/ providers and specialist physicians/specialist providers. Specialists want primary care providers to function at their highest level. The patient sees a specialist to receive a higher level of service, specific to the specialist's expertise, not because the insurance company would not pay the family practitioner to remove ear wax.

Third-party payers, like the government and insurance companies, use clever computer programs to reject bills from the doctor — as though the machines were pre-programed to reject a certain percentage. Although laws exist to prevent the rejection of so-called "clean claims" (i.e., perfectly coded documents), the profit is just too good to resist. Contending that ear wax removal was not medically necessary during Edward's office visit may be cost effective for third-party payers, but dismissive of the patient's needs.

Case Study – Clean Claim Documentation, Uncompensated Office Visit

Dr. Jones sees his patient for the management of multiple diseases, and submits a bill to the insurance company for the office visit. Despite the fact that the documents are perfectly coded, the insurance company denies the office visit charge a month later, suggesting that a copy of the doctor's office notes be sent for review. After two months and an additional seventy-five dollars in labor, Dr. Jones receives his ninety-six-dollar office visit payment.

Annual Wellness Examinations —

Once Every Twelve Months (Which Should Be Every Calendar Year)

Patients of all ages are encouraged to have a yearly wellness exam. Unlike an evaluation and management (E/M) for a specific medical problem or complaint, the annual wellness exam is intended "to develop or update a personalized prevention help plan to prevent disease and disability based on your current health and risk factors."[31] For people with Medicare and many private insurance policies, wellness exams are free. There is no co-pay or charge applied to a deductible. The rules for when you can have the exam, however, are flawed and should be corrected. Currently, federal rules dictate that the wellness exam must be performed *every twelve months*. If you had a wellness exam on November 14, 2012, then your next exam must be after November 14, 2013. If you are not able to schedule your next exam until December 17, 2014, then your next exam must be after December 17, 2015. If a practitioner does a good job of conducting annual wellness visits with his patients, the every-twelve-month rule will eventually make it impossible to complete a wellness exam for a given year. If the wellness exam is not completed, the provider will be labeled by the government and insurance companies as "not caring about the preventative needs" of patients. If you do not obtain a yearly wellness exam, your record may look as if "you do not care" about preventive health. Because private insurance plans follow government guidelines, we recommend that the Centers for Medicare and Medicaid Services (CMS) immediately change annual wellness exam rules from *once every twelve months* to *once every calendar year.*

Mixed Messages

Healthcare providers receive mixed messages from the government and insurance companies. On the one hand, medical providers are encouraged to see more patients, manage chronic diseases, and provide preventive care, while on the other hand are expected to document more in the health record. The system, however, seems to be set up to deter completeness. While such turmoil continues, we are facing a shortage of

---

31 Preventive visit & yearly wellness exams. (n.d.). Retrieved December 27, 2014, from http://www.medicare.gov/coverage/preventive-visit-and-yearly-wellness-exams.html

medical providers, as all Americans are federally mandated to have health insurance.

Imminent Solution: The Patient Advocate

Despite these obstacles, your ever-increasing participation in your healthcare story will allow you to control how your records are viewed and interpreted, avoid errors, and enhance the quality of your treatment. Your life is literally in your hands. Initially, this may sound intimidating. Enlightenment is empowering and forward-reaching. Learning how to look at your healthcare records will set you free. It's all there, right at your fingertips. Just turn the page to discover how.

Chapter 4

Managing Your Healthcare Data

The Patient Portal

Your first task in reviewing and managing your health record is to enroll in a patient portal. Your doctor's office will assist you in the process. Your patient portal is a secure, password-protected website that shows your personal health information, including test results and medical encounter notes (i.e., office visits, emergency room visits, hospital stays, etc.). Your patient portal gives you access to your health records and allows you to communicate with your healthcare professionals.

If your medical office does not offer a patient portal, it will soon. Patient portals are a consequence of the digitalization of health records. Your portal shares content with your doctor's electronic health record (EHR).

In order to enroll in the portal, you will require Internet access and an email address. You can open a free Gmail account with Google.com, and review your health records 24/7 from any computer, laptop, tablet or smartphone. If you do not have these devices, we recommend gaining access to your patient portal at a public library. The cost of your patient portal will be built into your medical provider's overhead expense. If your medical provider has not gone paperless yet, you may have to assume the customary costs of photocopying and printing. Although the techniques and suggestions offered in these pages can be implemented without the use of EHR's and patient portals, we strongly advise you to access the benefits of healthcare management through the computer.

One of the most salient issues that patients experience when confronted with reading their health records is a lack of understanding and knowledge of medical terminology. However, the wording is not as difficult as you may believe – and there are always dictionaries and online search engines. For example, an open sore above the outside of the right ankle might read,

"Stage II ulcer proximal to the right lateral malleolus." Fear not! Looking up the terms should instantly clarify meaning. Although you may be referencing Latin and Greek terms, the real challenge is understanding *how* the information is formatted. Learning a bit about medical, legal, and billing terminology will help decipher what you read.

Distinct Medical Provider-Patient Views

It is important to know that what you see on your patient portal and what your doctor sees in the EHR are different. What you see in the portal is not the same screenshot as what the doctor views in the office. Although the content may be the same, the formats are different. Your doctor's interaction with the EHR is designed to fulfill medical, legal, and billing requirements. Your online patient portal, by contrast, presents your information in a personalized, customer-friendly format.

Thus far, our data banks have been limited to the billing codes submitted by medical providers. Your office visits and/or procedures are billed with unique diagnostic codes that describe every disease and condition. Because your health records are now digitalized, the amount of information will explode from only a few billing data points to thousands of details recorded in electronic health records, producing a multitude of variables for evaluation — a functional network of comprehensive data. Now, virtually every piece of information — lab results, medications, diagnoses, the initial onset time of your condition, subsequent complications, etc. will be available for medical scrutiny. Welcome to the new age of medicine!

The Efficacy of "Break-the-Glass" Emergency Access

Patient portals are making provisions for so-called "break-the-glass" emergency access, which allows authorized personnel (e.g., emergency room staff members) to view your record — particularly in the event that you are unable to communicate. This feature of patient portals will, undoubtedly, save many lives, create peace of mind, and avert unnecessary expenditures associated with emergency room visits.

Consider this emergency scenario:

Stroke Victim's Medications Are Unknown

Joe goes to the grocery store and, while there, experiences confusion. The store manager calls an ambulance and stays with him until help arrives. Joe is rushed to the hospital, and undergoes a multitude of tests in the emergency room. Joe's altered mental state makes it hard for him to recall his medical conditions and medications. Because Joe's primary care doctor does not share the same EHR as the hospital, no one knows that Joe is taking warfarin, a blood thinner, as one of his prescriptions. Joe was diagnosed with a hemorrhagic stroke. His warfarin level was elevated, causing bleeding in his head. Because medical providers often work from scratch, their initial lack of knowledge about the blood thinner incurred additional expenses, and most significantly, could have cost Joe his life.

If Joe's electronic record interoperated with the emergency room's EHR, his medication list would have been readily available. The emergency medical technician (EMT) would have become aware of his warfarin use within moments of reaching the scene. "Break-the-glass" provisions, while not yet widely available, promise to help share knowledge until all EHR systems interoperate.

Access By Proxies and Other Personal Representatives

Via Privacy Rule 45 CFR §164.502(g), federal law confers your right and ability to delegate access to your chart to other people or "personal representatives".[32] This enables family members and friends to contribute and participate in the improvement of your health.

Consider these scenarios:

Young College Student Runs Out of Asthma Medication While Away From Home

Jack, a college sophomore studying for his final exams, finds his asthma inhaler to be empty with no refills. Although he is a long distance from home, he has no trouble getting a new inhaler. Jack has designated his mother as his personal representative. His mother is able to contact the medical office. Her communication results in a quick inhaler refill order. While Jack is home on break, his mother plans to show him how to use the portal to refill a medication on his own. For now, however, Jack has his nose in the books, and his mother is happy to help him. She appreciates the fact that she is able to coordinate his medical care.

Elderly Father, Living Independently, Has Diabetes and Visual Problems

Tom is in his mid 80's and has had diabetes for almost thirty years. He is on insulin, and has visual difficulties. Although he could elect to live in a nursing home, he prefers to live independently, in his own home. His daughter is a nurse, and though she lives a few states away, she does her best to help manage his medical care. When Tom's daughter calls

---

32 Your Medical Records. (n.d.). Retrieved November 24, 2014, from http://www.hhs.gov/ocr/privacy/hipaa/understanding/consumers/medicalrecords.html

him to ask about his doctor visit, he replies, "Doc said everything is OK." The daughter wishes that she could have more in-depth knowledge of her father's health status by viewing the doctor's note. Now, she can.

Personal Representatives and Privacy Concerns

Your health record "access log" will indicate who accessed your EHR and when. If you are concerned about privacy, you may not want to assign anyone as your personal representative. However, for the foregoing reasons, the benefits of doing so are vast. Remember, you can elect a personal representative in perpetuity (forever) or revoke that power after only a few minutes. You have the ability to direct your healthcare and make choices.

In choosing a personal representative, you will want to have a discussion about where you draw the line regarding privacy. For example, what is your personal representative permitted to discuss with friends and family? Remember, your personal representative has access to all of your health records.

Personalized Guidelines

For a time, you will only be able to access data reflecting *your* information, such as laboratory results and doctor's office notes. Soon, however, you will be able to compare your health data to information stored in huge databases, and access your health status in relation to others with similar conditions or difficulties. You will be able to ask questions and gain enhanced insight into your circumstances. With this heightened awareness, you and your doctor will be able to make decisions with an incredible level of insight.

Guidelines and recommendations are becoming very personalized. Thanks to the increasing prevalence of comprehensive databases, you will be able to predict outcomes based on your treatment approach. Decision options will soon become very user-friendly. Note how Amazon.com observes your purchases and offers similar or related items to complement or add to your personal cart. "If you liked that item, you might also enjoy these...." This approach will become increasingly more commonplace in healthcare. "If you have this disease, you might benefit from this treatment...or this one..." or, "You experienced a bad side effect from this medication. Other people who share your same conditions and had the same bad reaction found eighty-five percent success with the following treatment." Such personalized guidelines are not decades away. We predict that once we are able to correctly and efficiently manage our healthcare data, such services could emerge within five years.

Eliminating Errors

A British study found that when people review their online health records, 70% find at least one error or omission.[33] In the field of medicine, errors can and do occur. In 1999, the Institute of Medicine released "To Err Is Human: Building a Safe Health System," which brought attention to the forty thousand annual deaths in the United States caused by medical errors.[34] Ordering an MRI on the wrong shoulder is a waste of fiscal resources. Amputation of the wrong extremity, however, can cost you your leg!

EHR's Create New Opportunities for Error

EHR's create new possibilities for error. Let's explore two top reasons: 1. EHR's are new technology, and 2. systems are not yet interoperable (i.e., capable of seamlessly linking patient information across the healthcare network).

---

33 Pyper, C., Amery, J., Watson, M., & Crook, C. (2004). Patients' experience when accessing their on-line electronic patient records in primary care, *British Journal of General Practice*, p.40.
34 To Err is Human: Building a Safer Health System, by the Committee on Quality of Health Care in America and Institute of Medicine, © 2000

As with the introduction of any new innovation (let alone technology that creates a paradigm shift), there is a learning curve and mistakes are made. Worse yet, some mistakes may not be immediately recognizable. Going from paper charts to digital EHR systems is a huge leap for today's medical force. Younger doctors readily adopt EHR's, but 47.4 % of U.S. physicians are age fifty and over.[35] While younger physicians grew up using computers, much of the workforce was raised and trained to handwrite orders and notes. For people of any age, the introduction of electronic records has been a disruptive change in the practice of medicine. It will take time and effort to make EHR systems work efficiently and with minimal errors.

Lack of interoperability is perhaps the greatest contributor to errors in our healthcare system. With paper health records, information was fragmented into pieces of paper that were stored at various medical offices and hospitals. If you want to ensure quality, you must have *one* source of information. You cannot see three doctors and have three different medication lists! You can see three doctors, but your medication list has to be shared among all providers. In theory, EHR's eliminate fragmented data. Until they interoperate and share data, however, you are likely to have incomplete information stored in multiple databases. Currently, you can see a doctor and your records can be recorded in an electronic health record. You can then walk across the street and see another healthcare provider, only to start from scratch with another EHR system. Even if the EHR system is the same brand, the two offices may not be in the same service plan. This means that information cannot be shared. Interoperability magnifies problems associated with fragmented and/or inconsistent information.

In order to avert the pitfalls of reviewing and managing fragmented information, patients must stress the urgency of merging systems. Though better than paper medical charts, errors and mistakes – some of them fatal

---

35 A Survey of America's Physicians: Practice and Perspectives, by The Physicians Foundation, © 2012, 47.4% of U.S. physicians age 50 and over based on AMA Physician Master File source page 12 of Physicians Foundation report.

— can result from lack of continuity between EHR systems. Hopefully, tragedies won't occur before a government mandate is enforced.

We began using an EHR system in our private family practice in January 2012. Our staff exerted great effort in making the transition from written documentation to digitalized electronic health records. When our practice became part of the hospital system in 2013, we switched to another brand of EHR. In 2014, our hospital was purchased by a larger hospital system. This means that we will have to switch to yet another brand of EHR within the next year or two. None of these systems interoperate; hence, we must look at one computer screen and hand-type data from an old system into the new EHR. The potential for mistakes while learning an entirely new EHR system are minute when compared to the human error of typing information from one computer to another — and, then, another.

We know why EHR interoperability issues have occurred. Our situation is analogous to that of the videocassette recorder format wars — VHS versus Betamax - in the late 1970's and early 1980's. At the time, two separate formats were available for VCR's. Consumers were, therefore, faced with the question, "Which format should I buy?" Back then, due to the high cost of electronics, few people owned both versions. In much the same way, thousands of EHR systems entered the American healthcare market with the hope that the best would emerge. Though the number of EHR systems has decreased from thousands to hundreds, we still have interoperability issues. In fact, the situation is worse than VHS versus Betamax. Today, it is analogous to the ability to call a party only if he or she has your brand of phone and is within your service plan! Because of this break in communication, some EHR systems hold patient medical information in fragmented fashion — just like the nearly antiquated paper charts.

Within three to five years, we expect all of our systems to communicate with each other and interoperate because you, the patient, will not tolerate systems that do not communicate with each other. You cannot be expected to call an emergency room to find out whether it shares the same EHR system with your doctor — certainly not if you are unconscious or unable to speak! The Health Information Technology for Economic and Clinical Health Act (HITECH), formerly a Title XIII provision of the American Recovery and Reinvestment Act of 2009 (ARRA), promotes patient portals as part of meaningful use objectives. ARRA legislatively mandated the Office of the National Coordinator for Health Information Technology (ONC). The ONC is "the principle federal agency charged with coordination of nationwide efforts to implement and use the most advanced health information exchange to improve healthcare."[36] In other words, the federal government seeks to have all systems operating together, so as to share data. In the clinical world, this cannot happen quickly enough. Once you, the patient, complain, interoperability will be mandated.

We are already seeing patients with more than one patient portal — one from the family doctor, another from a specialist, and another from a specialty center. From a medical provider's point of view, no one is on the same page.

Ideally, your patient portal should link universally — to all of your doctors, not just to one EHR brand. Fragmenting your health data — whether in different written charts, different EHR systems, or different patient portals — is dangerous. Until systems interoperate, we urge you to choose a medical provider who shares an EHR system with others on your healthcare team (your family doctor, specialists, and/or urgent care provider, local emergency room/hospital) and find out whether their information will interface with your *one* patient portal, so that all of your information will be consolidated.

Structured Elements

We can print a document from one EHR system and scan it to another new system but, in all likelihood, it will not function as usable data. EHR systems focus on "structured elements" (i.e., information ready for data analysis). Often, the piece of information must be entered into a specific box within the EHR; otherwise, it is considered to be missing.

---

36 About ONC. (2014, June 14). Retrieved November 24, 2014, from http://www.healthit.gov/news-room/about-onc

Relationship to Partnership in Healthcare

We cannot emphasize too often that EHR/portal access will facilitate and shape your relationship with your medical provider. We realize that your newfound rights will also shape physician/medical provider behavior. For example, doctors who take a week or two to complete a medical note will be trained by their patients to finish work in a timely manner. In Chapter 9, we will address the physician perspective.

Aside from all of the technical aspects of synthesizing your healthcare data, such consolidation should, at the core, aim to facilitate a patient-provider relationship so as to support a partnership in healthcare. This involves personal knowledge sharing and genuine, concerned engagement on both sides. Learning how to build a meaningful relationship with your medical provider is the first step in mapping out a bright and healthy future. Turn the page, and empowerment shall be yours.

Chapter 5

Exercising Your Federal Rights with a Universal Pre-History

*D*octors and patients are sometimes entangled in a web of miscommunication in their face-to-face meetings. Your doctor may have a trying time in conducting a medical encounter due to the multitasks required by the EHR. The physician's focus is split between practicing medicine and functioning as a data entry clerk. The complexity of converting your story into the format of the EHR makes it likely that not all of your problem's details will be recorded in your health record. Consequently, when the details of your problem or chronic disease are incomplete, assessment and treatment plans are less likely to meet your needs.

Consider the following scenario:

Doctor-Patient Exchange —Lost in Translation:

Tabatha feels uncomfortable with her office visits. Her doctor is kind, but she senses that he does not understand what she is experiencing. She has severe rheumatoid arthritis (RA), which makes it difficult for her to do things that used to be simple. For example, she has trouble drying her hair with a blow dryer or using a curling iron.

When Tabatha reviews her health record, she discovers that her RA is listed as a diagnosis, but the record does not describe her difficulties in accomplishing daily tasks. She complains of her difficulties during medical encounters, but the details are never documented in her health record. She wishes that her doctor were on "her side," and that her limitations could be documented in her health record. We can show her how.

Entering information into your health record system is nothing new. Some EHR systems have the ability to work with an interactive touchscreen kiosk in the waiting room.[37] With such a system, you can verify your insurance as well as your demographic information (address, cellphone number, etc.). Such systems also allow you to document the reason for seeking medical attention. We expect such technology to become widespread. Waiting room kiosks and even patient portals will soon allow you to enter even more details about your condition. Remember, however, that you do not have to wait for technological advancement to enter information into your health record.

We suggest that you exercise your federal rights to amend your records and facilitate your healthcare *before* anything is written in your chart. You can do so by bringing a *Universal Pre-History* to your next doctor visit. Let us show you how to do it!

Universal Pre-History Documentation In Your EHR

We have assembled a universal pre-history form, designed to replicate the medical, billing, and coding needs of all EHR systems. At home, at your convenience, you can use this form to assemble your thoughts. With a little reflection, you can complete the form and bring it to your medical visit. When you arrive at your medical office, staff personnel have the option to enter information from your pre-history into the history section of the EHR. This process will allow you to fully express your concerns and problems *prior* to your provider entering the exam room. This will ensure that everything you need to express will be documented in your health record. The time your medical provider might spend asking and documenting these questions may take up most of your visit. Rather than spending your time answering basic questions and then watching your provider type answers into a computer, you will immediately be able to engage in a meaningful patient-provider dialogue.

---

37 Interactive Touchscreen Kiosks by Zivelo ™ (www.zivelo.com)

By completing a pre-history, you will facilitate the recording of your history, thus making your provider's job easier. The word "facilitate" comes from the French *faciliter* and the Latin *facilis*, meaning "to make easier" and "easy."

Your pre-history is your medical story, which creates the framework for all further action that medical providers will take on your behalf. The collaborative effort should be as seamless as possible. As mentioned, if your history is incomplete or wrong, your treatment will, most likely, be ineffective — and potentially dangerous.

Documenting your story in your health record – prior to your visit and prior to actually seeing your doctor — is the ultimate form of engagement in a medical partnership with your provider. You need not worry about forgetting details, or interruptions as you tell your story. The pre-history, therefore, bypasses previous lists that you may have prepared for medical visits, which were probably not designed to fit the EHR format.

An open dialogue is the hallmark of a productive patient-provider partnership. All of us have heard the expression, "communication is mostly non-verbal." The exact breakdown assigns 55% of communication to body language, 38% to the tone of the voice and 7% to the actual spoken words.[38] You can appreciate the importance of facial expressions, hand gestures, and body posture. We recommend that you have your side of the story documented quickly in the EHR, so that you and your medical provider can discuss details, encompassing all forms of communication. Specifically, you want to engage in eye-to-eye contact, which is difficult to do if your provider is multitasking with a computer! Your medical provider has extensive training and ability to help you. You just have to give him or her the chance. By assembling your concerns in advance and co-authoring your health record, you are enabling your medical provider to function at his or her highest level of expertise.

---

38 Thompson, J. (2011, September 30). Is Nonverbal Communication a Numbers Game? Retrieved December 11, 2014, from http://www.psychologytoday.com/blog/beyond-words/201109/is-nonverbal-communication-numbers-game

We encourage you to consider preparing a pre-history for your next medical encounter. Imagine dispensing with the burden of remembering the details of your concerns. Please review our universal pre-history, which can serve as a template. Then, as an example, see how it could apply to someone with right elbow pain.

Universal Pre-History

Cc: Chief complaint: "reason for your medical encounter"

HPI: History of Present Illness or Status of Chronic Disease

Location – where on body?
Quality – what does it look or feel like?
Severity – measurement with a number?
Duration – how long has it been occurring?
Timing – measurement of when the problem occurs?
Context – circumstances?
Modifying factors – what makes it worse or better?
Associated signs and symptoms – additional complaints?

(Status of Chronic Disease(s) can be used in place of the HPI or added to it)

ROS: Review of Systems

Constitutional - overall: energy level, weight loss?
Eyes – blurred or loss of vision?
Ears, nose, mouth, throat – sore throat?
Cardiovascular – chest pain?
Respiratory – shortness of breath?
Gastrointestinal – trouble eating or moving bowels?
Genitourinary – trouble urinating? Genital issues?
Musculoskeletal – joint or muscle pains or stiffness?

Integumentary – skin color changes, moles or rashes?
Neurologic – tingling, pain or trouble moving?
Endocrine – fatigue, increase in thirst?
Psychiatric – mood changes, feelings of depression or anxiety?
Hematologic/lymphatic – bruising or swelling?
Allergy/immunologic – seasonal allergies?

PFSH: Past Family Social History

Medication list
Allergies to medications
Prior surgery
Prior illnesses
Change in lifestyle
Change in family health history

(Free copies of these forms can be downloaded at
www.PatientAdvocacyInitiatives.org).

Here is how your pre-history might look if you had right elbow pain:

Pre-History – Right elbow pain example

Cc: Chief complaint :   *Right elbow pain*

HPI: History of Present Illness
1. Location – *Right elbow*
2. Quality – *Throbbing pain*
3. Severity – *pain 6/10*
4. Duration – *2 weeks*
5. Timing – *Constant pain*
6. Context – *Fell on ice at the park*

7. Modifying factors – *Better with rest and ibuprofen, hurts to move*

8. Associated signs and symptoms – additional complaints? *Fell a year ago doing the same thing and broke the same elbow.*

ROS: Review of Systems

Constitutional – *ok except for elbow*

Eyes – *ok*

Ears, nose, mouth, throat – *ok*

Cardiovascular – *no chest pain*

Respiratory – *no shortness of breath*

Gastrointestinal – *some stomach discomfort if ibuprofen is taken on an empty stomach*

Genitourinary – *ok*

Musculoskeletal – *just elbow*

Integumentary – *had bruise over elbow for few days after the fall*

Neurologic – *occasional numbness in my right ring and pinkie fingers*

Psychiatric – *ok*

Endocrine – *ok*

Hematologic/lymphatic – *bruising gone*

Allergy/immunologic - *ok*

PFSH: Past Family Social History

Medication list – *same as portal, see attached list, add ibuprofen 200mg one pill three times a day for past 2 weeks for pain*

Allergies to medications - *none*

Prior surgery – *none related*

Prior illnesses – *none related*

Change in something lifestyle: marital, occupation, smoking, alcohol, recreational drugs – *no change*

Change in family health history – *family doing well, no change*

Let's say "David" submits a Universal Pre-History at a doctor visit for his elbow pain. Upon arrival to the office, a staff member would scan David's pre-history as a document and enter it into a folder in the EHR. The content of his pre-history would be then entered into the History section of today's encounter note. David is exercising his federal rights to "request an amendment of his health record." He is facilitating his care by submitting a pre-history.

By submitting a pre-history, David is telling his story in his own words. He expects that the document will be scanned into his chart, and he hopes the content will be entered into the History section of today's office visit note. David can be sure that he is heard.

This is what the medical provider will see before he enters the room:

David Smith   DOB: 25oct1966
History:
cc: Right elbow pain

HPI: (Pre-Hx scanned) 48 year-old male with right elbow pain after falling on ice two weeks ago. Pain 6/10 constant throbbing. Increased pain with movement. Feels better with ibuprofen and rest. Friend had similar problem and needed a cast. This is the first medical encounter for this problem.
ROS: Overall feels ok except for right elbow pain, stomach discomfort when taking ibuprofen on an empty stomach and occasional tingling in right ring and pinkie fingers. Right elbow skin bruise resolved a few days after injury. No chest pain, no shortness of breath. Eyes/Ears/Nose/Throat/GU/Psych/Endo/Allergy: ok.
PFSH: You would see the entire medication list, plus:
Ibuprofen 200mg three tablets by mouth three times a day with food for pain and inflammation.

The remainder of PFSH would remain the same since there was no change)

Anyone with medical training can read this and understand what is going on. The astute healthcare professional may want to ask more questions about the stomach and the "tingling" in the fingers.

Personnel at the place of your medical encounter will know how to scan your pre-history into a "Pre-History" folder created for you in the EHR. Because everyone, from receptionist to provider, is used to working with the EHR, they will have little difficulty entering the content of your pre-history into the History section of today's office encounter note.

With a pre-history, you increase the efficiency of your medical visit. To facilitate your preparation for your medical visits, let's revisit the EHR format, in detail.

History
Cc:	***Chief Complaint***
HPI:	***History of Present Illness***
	(and/or "status of chronic disease")
ROS:	***Review of Systems***
PFSH:	***Past Family Social History***

Your history is one of three *key* components of a medical evaluation and management (history, examination, medical decision-making).[39] In addition to your chief complaint, your history includes your History of Present Illness (HPI), Review of Systems (ROS) and Past Family Social History (PFSH). The "Chief Complaint" states the problem, while the "History of Present Illness" describes details. "Review of Systems" surveys other parts of the body for any potential difficulties.

---

39 Professional Edition cpt® current procedural terminology 2014, © 2013, AMA Press, p. 6

Chief Complaint (cc:)

Your Chief Complaint should be a word or a short phrase to explain your problem. Its purpose: to provide the reason for your medical encounter. *Headache, sore throat, back pain,* and *fatigue* are examples. "Diabetes care" and "Hypertension care" are good chronic
care representations of a chief complaint. If you feel sick and cannot describe your problem with a term, then "I feel sick" is adequate. The details of your condition will be explained in the rest of your history.

History of Present Illness (HPI)

The History of Present Illness allows for the *where, what, and when* regarding your medical problem. *Location* represents anatomy, while *duration* describes how long you have had the problem, or when it first came to your attention. *Context* describes the circumstances in which the problem occurred. *Timing* describes how often the problem occurs, while *severity* measures how bad the problem is. *Severity* can often be described by using a number. The *severity* of pain, for example, can be given in the form of a number from "0" (no pain) to "10" (the worst pain ever). The *severity* of an asthma attack could be described by a home peak flow meter reading. *Quality* describes what the problem looks or feels like (e.g., the *hardness* of a breast mass, the *color* of a rash or the *throbbing* pain of an ingrown toenail.) *Modifying factors* describe what makes the pain worse or better. *Associated signs and symptoms* allow for additional complaints. This may include whether you were exposed to someone with an illness. It could also include whether this is the first time you sought medical attention for this problem. If not, then what happened?

Imagine that our friend David had been seen at an urgent care facility prior to seeing his primary care medical provider. His Associated signs and symptoms might look like this:

Associated signs and symptoms: *Seen at "MedWell" urgent care one week after the injury. Told no fracture per x-rays. Instructed to take*

Ibuprofen and see your primary care provider if you're if not better in two weeks.

It is tempting to write your problems in a list or paragraph form, but we recommend that you use the universal pre-history. Some EHR systems will have separate computer boxes or fields for each of the components that we have described. If you prepare written notes for your medical encounter in a non-EHR format, your medical staff member will not be able to enter your information into your health record prior to meeting with your provider. Your written material could be scanned into your record, but as previously mentioned, your document will likely be tucked in a compartment of your EHR that may never be reviewed. If a healthcare provider requires information about your history, he or she will look to the History section of your record. You want your information to be documented in the correct location.

Status of Chronic Disease versus History of Present Illness (HPI)

If your medical encounter concerns a chronic disease, then the HPI is not applicable. In its place, you should report the *status* of your condition or disease. If a person has Diabetes mellitus, for example, he could recount some of his home blood sugar readings, his last diabetic retinal exam, and an update on his exercise and dietary practices. If he had seen an endocrinologist (a doctor specializing in the treatment of disorders of the endocrine system, such as diabetes), he could describe what happened at the visit and what goals were made.

Review of Systems (ROS)

Review of Systems is a systematic inventory of your body and health systems. It ranges from *constitutional* ("overall, how do you feel?") to a checklist of *eyes, ears/nose/mouth/throat, cardiovascular, respiratory, gastrointestinal, genitourinary, musculoskeletal, integumentary (skin), neurologic, psychiatric, endocrine, hematologic/lymphatic, allergy/immunologic.*

A person experiencing shortness of breath may add "leg swelling" next to one of the categories, such as *lymphatic*. Shortness of breath with leg swelling is a red flag for medical personnel. Do not worry about your accuracy in picking the correct category to inventory your body. Simply doing your best will greatly aid your healthcare team.

Past Family Social History (PFSH)

Your *past, family,* and *social* history is the last part of your medical history. Your *past* history includes your current medications, any allergies to medications, foods or substances, past illnesses, past hospitalizations, surgeries, your immune status and your dietary status. Your *family* history is an inventory of the health of your family members. If a family member has a disease, such as diabetes or cancer, this is the area to record the information. Your *social* history records tobacco use, second-hand smoke exposure, alcohol use, recreational drug use, sexual orientation, level of education, occupation and employment status.

From a professional coding point of view, documentation requirements for billing reflecting this part of the history are surprisingly scant. A PFSH review of a *new* patient is considered *complete* if only <u>one</u> item from all three areas (*past, family* and *social history*) is recorded. This means that the maximum amount of PFSH credit can be attained by recording the following: medication, allergies, one example of a disease experienced by a family member, and whether or not you use tobacco. If you see your regular doctor (as an *established* patient) or go to the emergency room, then *complete* PFSH documentation is achieved if you record one item from only 2 of the 3 areas (*past, family* and *social history*).[40]

---

40 Medical Coding Training: CPC® 2014, © 2013 American Medical Association, p. 621

Billing and coding requirements give little incentive to the provider to document details in your health record. Fortunately, you can take it upon yourself to make sure that your medical problems are well-defined and documented.

You do not need to list every surgery you ever had in the prior history section. Your prior surgeries should already be documented in your health record. In our pre-history example of a person with right elbow pain, no surgeries were listed. If the person had undergone a previous right elbow operation, then the past surgery could have been listed in the past surgery section and/or in the context section of the HPI.

You do not have to write down your entire medication list prior to each medical visit. Next to PFSH in your pre-history, you could write "*same as in my portal.*" You should only do this if your portal and the EHR system in the medical office are linked. Then, you are looking at the same list. If you are taking Ibuprofen (as our hypothetical patient is doing for the elbow pain) you can write: "*same as portal, see attached list, add ibuprofen 200mg, one pill three times a day for past 2 weeks for pain.*" Because the medication list is one of the most prone to errors, we recommend that you print your medication list off of your portal and attach it to your pre-history. This is particularly crucial if you are scheduled to have a medical encounter with an office or facility that is not interfaced with your patient portal.

Due to the advent of electronic health records, you will likely find your PFSH area to be nearly blank. As a priority, we recommend that you ensure the accuracy of your medication and allergy lists. Over time, work with your healthcare provider and staff members to build additional components to this part of your documented history.

Universal Pre-History Focus on History (HPI/status, ROS, PFSH)

One could argue that your pre-history is limited only to the history component of your medical encounter. Recall that the documentation requirements of your medical encounter include three key components: history, exam, and medical decision-making. We appreciate this argument, but want to point out that *everything* in your health record is history, once the encounter is over. Your ability to participate in your care through federal rights supporting a pre-history is powerful. Your intervention has the ability to reflect everything that has happened to you, as well as direct where your care will go next. To see how your pre-history can apply to you, let's explore the application of the pre-history.

Chapter 6

Universal Pre-History Applications

*I*n this chapter, we will explore how to apply a pre-history to various situations that may pertain to you or someone you love. We will start with seemingly straightforward problems and then, discuss situations where the problem is unspecific or unknown.

Pre-History and the Straightforward Problem

Our previous example of right elbow pain shows a straightforward pre-history. The History of Present Illness (HPI) describes pertinent details of the condition relating to the where, what and when. The Review of Systems (ROS) offers information about stomach upset that is associated with the use of ibuprofen. The Past Family Social History (PFSH) includes the addition of ibuprofen to the medication list.

When a problem is straightforward, it is tempting to skip using a pre-history, but would you have remembered to include the upset stomach? And what about the tingling in the fingers? If you did mention it, do you think it would have been documented in your history?

Pre-History and a Complex Problem

"Trouble breathing" or "pains in the chest when walking" are not straightforward. In such cases, your prepared history (cc, HPI, ROS, PFSH) becomes tremendously valuable to your healthcare provider. Details regarding the various questions in the pre-history, such as "when did the problem first start" and "what makes your problem better or worse?" are likely to make your head spin while you're in the medical office. Though you may have some difficulty coming up with answers for the universal pre-history, we believe it is worth your time. We are quite certain that without a pre-history, you would spend most of your healthcare visit trying to answer these same questions. Worse yet, your health record probably would not be as complete without your pre-history.

Pre-History and Multiple Problems

If you are a patient with multiple symptoms and conditions, you might believe that you could complete multiple pre-history forms. Electronic health record (EHR) systems, however, cannot accommodate the entry of multiple pre-history forms. EHR's are formatted to meet billing and coding rules, and these rules allow for only <u>one</u> history (HPI/ROS/PFSH) per encounter. To address multiple chief complaints, you need to combine the multiple problems into one pre-history.

Imagine if someone had a sore throat, an ingrown toenail, and an abnormal mammogram. It is tempting for a medical provider to say, "Let's take care of one of these today and you can come back another day." We ask, "What would you take care of today?" Would you take care of the abnormal mammogram and forget you ever heard about the sore throat or ingrown toenail? What if the sore throat is due to *Streptococcus pyogenes*? Strep throats have the ability to develop into rheumatic fever and possibly cause rheumatic heart disease. Query: how can patients be expected to prioritize or subordinate serious conditions to others, and why should they have to choose?

If you organize your problems with the universal pre-history and give it to a member of the medical staff when you arrive at your visit, we anticipate that you will have a productive encounter. After all, in such a scenario, you want the focus of your visit to be about "what is 'abnormal' about my mammogram?" *and* "what should we do next?" *and* "what can I do about this ingrown toenail" *and* "should I be concerned about my sore throat?"

We believe that competent medical care occurs when a history is discussed and documented. Great care emerges when deeper questions are asked and medical decision-making occurs. Currently, the medical interview often dwells on basic information with only moments of deep engagement — an inefficient approach. Your pre-history helps to ensure the basics, so that you and your provider can work beyond your history.

If you do not construct a pre-history, you may impede the quality of your care. For example, we recommend that you do not bring up a new chief complaint at the end of the visit. Such "by the way" complaints can be highly disruptive in a medical setting. With knowledge of the required format for the history component of your medical encounter, you can see why. At the end of the visit or at the checkout counter, a "by the way" additional chief complaint is an EHR nightmare. Either the provider must dismiss the complaint as having no significance, or he must re-open the health record and add to the history: *when did it start, what makes it better/worse, etc.* Avoid "by the way" complaints by organizing your thoughts in advance of your medical encounter and inform the medical staff of your problems early in your visit. We believe that the pre-history best accomplishes this objective.

Pre-History and Multiple Chronic Diseases or Conditions

Multiple chronic diseases or conditions pose some of the same challenges as multiple new problems: the EHR can accommodate only one history. In the case of chronic diseases, the History of Present Illness (HPI) component of the history is replaced with the *Status of Chronic Disease.*

If you have Diabetes mellitus, hypertension, high cholesterol and hypothyroidism, instead of completing an HPI, you would comment on each of the diseases/conditions. Your status might look like this:

Status of Chronic Diseases/conditions:

Diabetes: *fasting glucometer readings around 120. I check my feet daily and have no sores. I saw the eye doctor last month and the eye exam showed no problems.* **Hypertension**: *My home blood pressures are around*

130/80, I do not get lightheaded when I stand up. **Cholesterol, Thyroid** *and other conditions: I take all of my medication as prescribed and experience no bad effects from them. I exercise at the gym three days a week. I do 20 minutes of cardio on the elliptical machine and then work out on the weight machines.*

If a person has a problem with a medication, the status might look like this:

Cholesterol: *I had to stop taking my statin medication a month ago. My legs ached so bad that I could not get out of a chair. My legs feel better now.*

Once again, such scenarios highlight the advantages of completing a pre-history in advance of your next medical visit. It is important that you deliver this information and it is crucial that it is documented in your health record. Proper use of a pre-history ensures documentation.

Pre-History: Multiple Chronic Diseases and Multiple Problems

If you have multiple chronic conditions, you will have new problems emerge over time. Logging your information into the universal pre-history means that you will have to complete an HPI for the new problem(s) and also account for the status of each of your chronic diseases or conditions. EHR systems do not allow for multiple history forms (HPI, PRS, PFSH). All of the information you need and want to offer at a medical encounter must fit on one pre-history form.

Pre-History and the Unknown Diagnosis

As a patient, the most frustrating medical problem is the one that no one can figure out. Perhaps, you have a condition that has eluded detection? Perhaps, you have symptoms that have not yet presented themselves so as to allow for an accurate diagnosis? You may have been given a generalized or non-specific diagnosis, such as "abdominal pain" or "back pain" or "fatigue." If this ever applies to you, then you want to prepare your pre-history with particular attention to your last medical encounter. Was your last HPI documented accurately? Was the content appropriate? In other words, is there something missing or incorrect in your medical story? Was anything found to be abnormal on physical examination? Were any tests abnormal, thus ruling out another problem? In general, you want to clarify your observation and document it as part of the *status* of your condition.

Arguably, the most important question in preparing your pre-history is, "What do you understand about your condition?" The answer is rarely documented. Imagine that a person with cancer does not understand the nature of his condition; imagine a personal representative who wants everything done for her father, but does not realize that treatment is no longer indicated.

The worst scenario in healthcare occurs when your assessment and expectations deviate from your doctor's. If you sense that you and your provider are not on the same page, your pre-history will help you to remedy the situation.

When it comes to your healthcare and an unknown or uncertain diagnosis, you want to be heard. By reviewing your record after your medical encounter, you can verify that your questions, concerns, and needs were understood. You should then draw your attention to the assessment and plan parts of the encounter note. The assessment should define "what is known so far about your condition" while the plan should outline "what needs to be done." As you understand what is going on, you will be able to participate more intensely in shared decision-making with your medical provider.

Despite all of your effort, your condition may continue to remain a mystery. At the least, you now know how to express your symptoms. You also know how to review your records on your portal. Working with your provider, we hope you are able to find a definitive diagnosis along with an effective treatment.

Review your record before and after medical encounters

Whether you prepare a written pre-history or not, it is best that you review your health record before and after medical encounters. This is the most valuable advice that we can give you. Checking for proper content and accuracy makes *you* your own best patient advocate.

If you find errors, you will assist in correcting them. If you find. inaccuracies, then you will offer clarity. You are not expected to practice medicine, but to best represent yourself and your medical story. Remember, your health record is a documentary of your life in health and disease. It is your story.

Preparing and implementing a written pre-history can seem overly aggressive, until you consider the alternative problems that are likely to occur. Come with us to the next chapter. Let's address what patients really want before we open Pandora's Box.

Chapter 7

In Search of Empathy

*P*atients want many things as part of their healthcare experience. We believe that *empathy* is one of the most important components (in fact, the essence) of the patient-provider relationship. Patients want doctors/medical providers and everyone on the healthcare team to empathize with their problems, so as to provide the best healthcare possible. In a Cleveland Clinic survey, "82% of patients highlighted doctor empathy as being important. Significantly, many patients were willing to overlook common grievances, such as waiting to get an appointment with their doctor or protracted wait times in the office to see the doctor."[41]

The word *empathy* was coined in 1858 by German philosopher and physician Rudolf Hermann Lotze, M.D., Ph.D. when the Greek *empatheia* was translated to German.[42] [43] According to Dictionary.com, empathy in medicine means to "direct identification with, understanding of, and vicarious experience of another person's situation, feelings, and motives."

Empathy differs from sympathy, in that sympathy acknowledges another person's hardships and calls for offerings of comfort and assurance.[44] Empathy, on the other hand, allows medical professionals to understand what their patients are *feeling*, enabling the healthcare provider to view a given situation from the patient's perspective.

In the context of patient care, "empathy is predominantly a *cognitive* attribute, which involves an *understanding* of experiences, concerns, and

---

41 The Most Common Gripes Patients Have About Their Doctors. (2014, January 17). Retrieved December 27, 2014, from huffingtonpost.com
42 Empathy. (n.d.). Retrieved December 27, 2014, from www.dictionary.com
43 Debate exists as to whether Philosopher Rudolf Lotze or Psychologist Edward Titchener coined the term "empathy" (see cultureofempathy.com)
44 Empathy vs. Sympathy. (n.d.). Retrieved December 27, 2014, from diffen.com

perspectives of the patient, combined with a capacity to *communicate* this understanding, and an <u>*intention to help.*</u>"[45] [46]

It is tempting to think of empathy as esoteric. Of interest, however, is the fact that empathy has been defined with enough rigors to be scientifically validated. A physician's level of empathy can be measured when taking care of patients. Study results demonstrate better healthcare for you when your doctor experiences high levels of empathy.

The Jefferson Scale of Empathy (JSE) has become a validated and reliable measure of physician empathy. Studies have correlated higher physician empathy scores with better clinical outcomes, and lower empathy scores with poor outcomes. When physicians show high empathy and care for patients with Diabetes mellitus, for example, there are fewer hospitalizations, lower A1c values (reflecting better long-term blood glucose levels), and lower LDL levels (lower "bad" cholesterol). As you can imagine, patients were also more satisfied with their healthcare.

We recommend that you do everything you can to encourage and evoke empathy in anyone who cares for you. Remember, someone with sympathy will feel sorry for you. In contrast, a person with empathy will seek to gain your perspective, so as to understand your situation. You want your medical provider to experience empathy when caring for and treating you!

Take a moment and experience empathy, as you consider the role of your physician/medical provider. Due to the recent introduction of EHR systems, your provider is likely to feel rushed to ask you basic questions and enter the responses into the computer. Your provider is also likely to feel pressured by a multitude of tasks required by the EHR. Does this invite high levels of empathy?

---

45 Hojat, M. (Speaker) (2014, October 27). Empathy In the Realm of Evidence-Based Medicine. *Annual Meeting of the American Osteopathic Association.* Lecture conducted from Center for Research in Medical Education and Health Care, Department of Psychiatry and Human Behavior, Sidney Kimmel Medical College at Thomas Jefferson University, delivered in Seattle, Washington.

46 Hojat, M. (2007). *Empathy in Patient Care: Anticedents, Developments, Measurement, and Outcomes* (p. 80). Philadelphia, Pennsylvania: Center for Research in Medical Education and Health Care, Jefferson Medical College.

Whenever you can, you want to flip the approach to your medical story. You are the expert on what is happening to you. The scientific name of your condition or the scientific reason for its existence may be difficult for you to understand, but you can leave that to the doctor. You, however, know what is happening to you and how you are affected. By reviewing your records before and after medical encounters, you can check your medical story for accuracy and content. Is your story properly documented? Will medical providers understand your situation by reading your health record? Will your documented medical story evoke empathy? If this is not the case, we recommend infusing your perspective into your health record with a pre-history.

Nothing About Me Without Me

"Nothing about Me Without Me" is a fitting blurb for patient advocates. It was described in a 1998 psychiatric journal in support of patient empowerment.[47] Now, the slogan represents your ability to control your part of the patient-provider relationship. Though the slogan directly applies to what is documented in your health record, it quickly expands medical decision-making to shared decision-making. This occurs when the doctor *and* you decide what is going on and what to do next. Like empathy, shared decision-making fosters improved healthcare and better outcomes. Studies show that patients experience greater satisfaction and higher quality healthcare when they actively participate in decisions that affect them.[48] [49] Shared decision-making allows all of us, as patients, to work with our medical providers in a healthcare partnership.

---

47 Nelson, G., et al. (1998). 'Nothing about me, without me': Participatory action research with self-help/mutual aid organizations for psychiatric consumers/survivors. *American Journal of Community Psychology*.

48 Berwick, D. (n.d.). What 'Patient-Centered' Should Mean: Confessions Of An Extremist. Retrieved December 27, 2014, from healthaffairs.org

49 Barry, M. , et. al. (1995). Patient Reactions to a Program Designed to Facilitate Patient Participation in Treatment Decisions for Benign Prostatic Hyperplasia. *Medical Care, 33* (8), 771-782.

Chapter 8

Pandora's Box

Digitalization of Medical Records —
The Government Already Opened Pandora's Box

*I*n classical Greek Mythology, the god Prometheus stole fire from heaven and gave it to man. Zeus, king of the gods, was not pleased. However, rather than cast instant wrath, he gave a box (in the original story, "jar") to Pandora as a wedding gift. Pandora was about to marry Epimetheus, the brother of Prometheus. With the gift came instructions *to never open it*. Unbeknownst to Pandora, the box (jar) contained all of the evils of the world. Driven by curiosity (a trait instilled in her by the gods), Pandora opened the box and evil spread throughout the world.[50]

Opening your health records may feel like opening Pandora's box, but that box has *already* been opened due to the digitalization of health records and federal law. Whether you enroll in a patient portal or not, your records are in a digital database. We understand that our records have to be in databases, so as to allow for better tracking and management of healthcare. While databases are necessary, new issues arise in regard to patient rights. Let's expose some of the disruptive problems that EHR's can cause, and then we will address more severe consequences.

Your First Look at Your Health Records

When you first look at your personal health records, you may become frustrated, upset or disappointed. The terminology used to describe

---

50 Athanassakis, Hesiod: Theogony, Works and Days, Shield, 2004 The Johns Hopkins University Press

you in your health record may be cold and impersonal. Worse yet, your medical story might not look like you. Some information may not be accurate, while important details may be missing. We do not believe that your curiosity will unleash the evils in Pandora's box. Rather, seeking knowledge and understanding will allow you to achieve better health.

Seeing What the Doctor Writes About You

For our entire careers, only a few of our patients have ever read what we have written about them. Moving forward, they will be able to read every word. We see this new era of transparency as perhaps the most intriguing manifestation of HIPAA. We expect many of you to be very curious to read what your medical provider has written about you.

When you read your health record, does it reflect what occurred during the medical encounter? Were actions documented that did not occur? Were discussions documented that were not addressed, or was not enough written to capture what actually did occur during the visit? For a better understanding, let's look at some potential problems caused by EHR systems.

Templates

EHR's allow for the creation of *templates*. A template allows for a few clicks to populate fields with paragraphs or pages of information. Templates are more than time savers. Without templates, a medical provider may forget to add important information. Sometimes, however, a template may add too much information. A doctor may perform a detailed examination of one knee, but the template may indicate that both knees were examined.

Copy Forward

Errors in documentation can also come from the EHR "copy forward" function. Copy forward allows information from a previous encounter to be placed in today's note. If you saw the doctor and were found to have a heart murmur, the doctor may copy forward your examination from a previous visit to today's note in order to capture the murmur description. If however, you had an erythematous (red) tympanic membrane (eardrum) during the previous visit, then "copy forward"would show that you have a red eardrum today, too. If you see something written in your health record that was not done or did not occur, then be aware that it could be an unintended consequence of a template or copy forward function. Notify your office with a message through the portal to highlight the error. Your provider should be able to edit the note in order to correct the error.

Insufficient Documentation

Sometimes, the documentation will not support what was discussed or occurred at the medical encounter. You may have discussed three problems, but find only one or two are documented in your record. In this instance, do not assume that your doctor does not care about you or did not understand your problems. The doctor may have been so focused on your story, that he did not have time to document what you said. If your health record does not document your story to your satisfaction, you could send a note to your doctor, asking for a correction. After the visit, however, you may encounter problems as you instruct the provider to add information to your health record.

Simple tasks (such as "it was my left shoulder, not my right shoulder") can be easily edited and corrected. This may be of immediate importance if you are about to get a MRI of the wrong shoulder.

Attempts to add detailed descriptions to a medical encounter that has already occurred, however, can be problematic. For example, "I had shortness of breath and chest pain. Please add it to my last note." In nearly all cases, this will not and cannot be documented as part of a previous medical encounter. Were these issues discussed at the visit? Was appropriate action taken at the encounter? Most of the time, your "corrections" are meant to clarify what you experienced at the medical encounter. To most efficiently correct detailed information, you should prepare for the next encounter with a pre-history.

Inaccurate Information

Occasionally, information is added into the wrong person's health record. A report for the Agency for Healthcare Research and Quality found that information is entered in the wrong chart two percent of the time per week.[51] We understand this to mean that for every medical provider, two patients per week have information mistakenly entered into their health record. If you do not have Diabetes mellitus, but now find it as one of your diagnoses, it may have been mistakenly entered into your health record. You can respond by contacting the office and asking for a correction.

Finding and Preventing Medication List Inaccuracies/Errors

You should look at your health record before and after every medical encounter, paying close attention to your medication list. If your doctor told you to double the dose of your blood pressure medication, your medication list must show that your dose is now twice as strong as it was. If the change has not been made, you have to ensure that it's corrected by sending an electronic message via your portal.

The Agency for Healthcare Research and Quality report was constructed from a 2012 database, where workers in medical offices throughout the United States answered surveys. The report shows that medication lists are not updated in seven percent of patients seen daily.[52] This report was constructed from a 2012 database. In this study, sixty-two percent of the medical practices in the study had EHR systems, and

---

51 Medical Office Survey on Patient Safety Culture: 2012 User Comparative Database Report, prepared for the Agency of Healthcare Research and Quality, U.S. Department of Health and Human Services, May 2012, p. 28
52 Medical Office Survey on Patient Safety Culture: 2012 User Comparative Database Report, prepared for the Agency of Healthcare Research and Quality, U.S. Department of Health and Human Services, May 2012, p. 30

thirteen percent were implementing them. We would like to believe that as EHR use increases, medication lists will be updated in nearly all medical visits. When a medical provider uses an EHR and sees a patient, he or she has the option of looking at the medication list and clicking a "medication reconciliation" button. Whether your doctor checks your medication list or not, you should always check it before and after a medical encounter.

In addition, you should learn what your medications are for. To help you, ask your medical provider to write the *purpose* of each of your medications in the instructions. For example, *Amoxicillin 500mg, one pill by mouth with food, three times a day, for ten days for sinusitis.* If the instructions did not include "for sinusitis," you wouldn't easily be able to decipher the reason for taking the medication. "For sinusitis" also makes it clear to any medical professional why you are taking the medication. If Amoxicillin is still present on your medication list four months later, someone in your medical office will be quick to question whether it should be taken off of your current list.

Some medications can be taken for more than one reason. Lisinopril, for example, is a medication to treat hypertension. Besides being used for high blood pressure, it is also used to treat heart failure. Consider the following medication list:

Baby Aspirin 81mg one tablet by mouth daily
Amlodipine 5mg one by mouth daily
Lisinopril 10mg one by mouth daily
Pravastatin 40mg one by mouth at bedtime

The medication list does not tell you much, other than to take the medication once a day by mouth. Compare this list to the more descriptive list:

Baby Aspirin 81mg one tablet by mouth daily for heart disease
Amlodipine 5mg one by mouth daily for hypertension
Lisinopril 10mg one by mouth daily for hypertension and heart failure
Pravastatin 40mg one by mouth at bedtime for cholesterol

The second list makes it clear why you are taking each medication. These instructions are not only recorded in your health record, but also on the instructions on the side of your prescription bottles. If you read the list first, you might think that the patient is mistakenly taking two blood pressure pills. This might tempt someone to get rid of the Lisinopril.The second list identifies Lisinopril as being taken for both hypertension and heart failure. We recommend you work with your medical providers to document the reason for taking your medication, and include it in the prescription instructions, so that it appears on the side of prescription bottles.

Can I See Everything in My Health Record?

Despite having a federal right to view your health record, we find five instances in which you may not see them. They include: technical development issues, provider authorization, worker's compensation notes, motor vehicle accident records, psychotherapy notes and if the provider believes that the notes contain information that may harm you.

It is easy to forget that electronic health records are new to medical care. Some systems may only allow you to see blood tests and radiology results because they are still in the process of load-testing their network. Once the network is shown to support a large number of people, the patient portal will be expanded to include the notes from office, emergency room and hospital visits. If you are not able to see your health record, expect to do so soon.

In order for you to see a note from an office visit, the doctor must first "authorize" the note. If the doctor or medical provider does not authorize the note, it will be considered unfinished and will stay hidden from your view. Doctors authorize the note by clicking a button.

We realize that technology takes time to implement and we understand that doctors and medical professionals must authorize and electronically "sign" the note from an encounter before you are allowed to see it. We are willing to argue, however, that you *should* be able to see your health records that pertain to worker's compensation and mental healthcare.

If you are involved in an injury while at work, your care will be paid for by a worker's compensation claim. It is important to know that worker's compensation is HIPAA exempt. You do not have the right to view health records that pertain to worker's compensation.

Because worker's compensation claims are HIPAA exempt, you do not have a right to review your health record before and after medical encounters. You also do not have a right to amend your record with a universal pre-history. We encourage providers of worker's compensation care to allow you to view your records. They should welcome your review and participation.

How can you be an advocate of your healthcare if you are not permitted to see your health records relating to a worker's compensation case? What if an error occurred in your health record? What if a diagnosis of *knee pain* (719.46) was mistakenly documented, and you actually had *wrist pain* (719.43)? What if you had both wrist and knee pain, but the medical provider only documented knee pain? Because the treatment is tailored to your return to work, such omissions could impact your ability to perform your occupation.

If a medication is prescribed as part of your worker's compensation care, we highly recommend that the records be shared with your primary care provider. Unbeknownst to your worker's compensation company, you may have a condition that could be worsened by the medication. Keeping some of your health records with one provider and a separate set of records with another defeats the purpose of electronic health records and exposes you to harm. Similar restrictions apply to most motor vehicle accident records. This issue may depend on local laws.

The Standards for Privacy of Individually Identifiable Health Information, also known as the "Privacy Rule," was created so as to implement the requirements of HIPAA 1996. The Privacy Rule states that you do not have a right to access psychotherapy notes taken by a mental health professional.[53]

Whether a patient should be able to see mental health notes is debatable. Professionals are concerned about how patients would react if they read what was written about them. Consider the next story:

Carla was in the hospital for a blood clot in her leg. She was receiving all of the appropriate medication and was expected to go home the next day. She expressed a sudden feeling of depression while in the hospital. Upon further discussion, she revealed details regarding her brother's suicide some time ago. Her doctor documented a full page of details and consulted a psychiatrist. The next morning, the doctor asked Carla about the psychiatric consultation. "He told me to take some pills. I saw him a few minutes ago," she explained. At the nurses' station, Carla's doctor met with the psychiatric physician. When asked about Carla, the psychiatrist responded that she was depressed and would benefit from medication. When asked about the brother's suicide, the psychiatrist looked stymied; and when questioned about whether he had read the notes in the chart or discussed the topic with Carla, it became apparent he had not. Worse yet, the request for a psychiatric consultation read, "Please read today's progress note." It was clear that he had no idea of her story.

If Carla had the ability to see her mental health notes, she would have gained better insight into her care. She potentially could have recognized the lack of understanding and been given the opportunity to discuss her needs. By law, however, she cannot review these notes.

While the Privacy Rule defines "psychotherapy notes,"   we   fear that the use of any psychiatric diagnostic code could someday block you from viewing your records. From a Patient Advocacy standpoint, we should closely watch the application of the Privacy Rule. Should Carla have been able to see her chart? Whom are we trying to protect?

---

53 Standards for Privacy of Individually Identifiable Health Information (The Privacy Rule), http://www.hhs.gov/ocr/privacy/hipaa/understanding/consumers/medicalrecords.html

We struggle to define situations in which patients should not be able to see their own records. Should Grandpa be barred from seeing his records if his cancer returns? Should someone not be told that they have an aneurysm in their brain? How would you feel if you were suddenly barred from seeing your health records?

In our years of practicing medicine, we find trouble when the patient and the doctor think they are on the same page – when, in fact, they are not. Difficulties are compounded as the partnership diverges. For the elderly man who has a weak heart, we feel that it is acceptable to discuss an ejection fraction of 14%.[54] The approach of the provider can be optimistic and hopeful, while also being realistic. In a country where patients need more information about their healthcare, we are guarded about blocking information.

Fear of Test Results

We know what it is like to review test results of our patients. Unfortunately, we also know what it is like to review test results of family members and ourselves. We, too, have worked the computer with one hand, clicking to reveal the results, while covering our eyes with the other. For the female who wishes to be pregnant, a *positive* result is a cause for jubilation. What if, however, the CT scan describes a lesion that is highly suspicious for cancer?

In 1976, the Federal Drug Enforcement Agency (FDA) approved the first home pregnancy test kit.[55] Without requiring a doctor's order, you can purchase and perform a long list of kits that can test for urinary tract infections to human immunodeficiency virus (HIV). Though currently

---

54 Left Ventricular Ejection Fraction (LVEF) is like a "horsepower" measurement of the heart. This value can be found on an echocardiogram, a nuclear stress test or a cardiac catheterization. Normal is around 55%. At 12% or less, it is difficult to get out of a chair.
55 A Timeline of Pregnancy Testing, A Thin Blue Line: The History of the Preganancy Test Kit, presented by The Office of the National Institutes for Health (NIH) History. retrieved 18jan2015 http://history.nih.gov/exhibits/thinblueline/timeline.html

under government restrictions, tests are available to test you for genetic links to disease.

How will you react when you see "abnormal" printed next to one of your lab results?

Next to blood tests, for example, a reference range is listed. You can think of it as the normal range, but this definition does not always apply. A test result could be out of reference range and be normal for you. As you get used to seeing your laboratory values, we caution against over reaction to a test that is labeled as abnormal. This is particularly important if you see the result before anyone else.

Some people argue that you should not be able to see any laboratory results until your medical provider reviews them. Due to recognizing the patient as a client, however, we anticipate that *all* test results will become available to you once they are performed and uploaded into the EHR system.

When a patient is found to have a significant abnormality, like the finding of cancer, we prefer to have a face-to-face encounter. The telephone is not a good enough means of communication. We want you to have a strong bond with your medical provider so to best handle any abnormality.

Fear of Hackers

Some people fear that having or accessing their online health records will enable nefarious Internet hackers. Could your information be captured and used without your knowledge or with criminal intent? Without a doubt, the answer is yes. Electronic health records are in databases similar to the credit card databases that were compromised at major retail stores. In the past, it was more difficult to access private medical information. Someone would need to physically break into a medical office in order to illegally view a health record. Now, anyone in the world can try to overcome security protocols and gain access to your medical file, which has more personal, identifying information than probably any other single record of yours. Worse yet, hacking can be done with anonymity!

Electronic health record information needs to be protected at all levels from government on down to institutions and even to individuals. Advanced security technology is in place to deter snooping and hacking; but it takes constant updating to maintain and enforce security protocols. It will be an ongoing challenge for everyone in the information age. As an individual patient, though, it is your responsibility to check your records to detect potential tampering and ensure accuracy – just like you would your credit card or bank statement.

In addition to monitoring your records, it is important for you to take security precautions. You should change your password on a regular basis and not share it with anyone, but a trusted individual. Remember, your personal representatives will have their own passwords to enter your record.

Criminal Activity

You must beware of criminals who might send you requests for information. If someone needs your information, they can get it by contacting your doctor.

Consider this hypothetical email:

Mrs. Jones, we are having trouble processing your last blood test. If we do not do it correctly, you could be charged $350. We need information contained in your health record to dismiss the charge. Please send us your username and password. Be on guard for criminal activity, and do not share your username and password.

Fear of Being Watched

Some people fear that the use of a patient portal will enable the government to view personal information. The government *already* has the right to view and use data generated by your health records. For research purposes, your information is "de-identified" meaning that the information is stripped of your identity. Because such information can be used to track dangerous diseases and infections, it serves an important public health need. We see no problem with the government's right and responsibility to protect our society, so we are not worried about them watching our data. We do, however, have concerns about the permanency of your digital record. The following questions can, potentially, arise:

Is it necessary to save all of the medical history forever?

Do healthcare providers "pre-judge" a patient who has a documented medical encounter that showed intoxication of alcohol? Or, showed a positive test for an illegal recreational drug? What if the patient was sexually abused? – What if all of these things happened 15 years ago?

Should we treat medical charts the way we do criminal records and block certain past items that may affect the way a patient is treated in the present?

Do patients have the right to "put the past in the past" and have certain parts of their no-longer-relevant medical history deleted? If so, which items and when?

Every Word is Saved Forever

Doctors take an oath that specifically addresses the confidential nature of the physician-patient relationship. You should be able to confide in your doctor and all medical providers. Now, with so many details recorded and kept forever, you need to carefully consider what you are sharing.

As a society of citizens, we need to be vigilant about the consequences of digital records. Are we ready to commit every piece of data to our healthcare timeline? Will we need to establish rules so to define when some parts of our health records can be deleted?

Consider the following scenarios:

A young adult is concerned that he may have been exposed to a sexually transmitted disease. He goes to the clinic and requests testing.

Years later, his new wife becomes his personal representative. She reviews the details of the encounter years ago that addressed his possible STD infection.

Imagine a patient who is upset because a medication prescription is not properly refilled. What if he submits a message through his portal with inflammatory language? Will this message stay in his file forever? Will it make him appear to be a disruptive patient? What if he was perfectly justified in using such strong words? What if he regrets what he wrote?

To automatically delete all records after five years is not the answer. A person with cancer or a heart attack will want all the details available. Additionally, as our society exploits genetic medicine, specific medical details may be important for future family generations. We anticipate that these issues will be the subject of much debate in the future. For now, if you recognize a need to delete information in your record, you should act quickly. We recommend talking with your provider or using a pre-history at another encounter to "set the story straight."

With all of our technological advancements, we will have to work diligently to set up guidelines for the use of patient information. Despite the benefits of digitalization, there will be unintended consequences that will require our attention. Query: At what point in the future will a video camera be a standard method of recording medical encounters? Are we ready for that level of transparency? Everyone has to be part of the discussions in which laws and guidelines are created to control this information.

Pandora's Box has been open since HIPAA 1996. The dangers associated with the digitalization of your health records have already been unleashed. Due to the adoption of EHR systems, however, we are just beginning to face the consequences. We urge everyone to watch these issues closely.

Please join us in our next chapter, as we reach out to doctors and all medical providers.

Chapter 9

A Message to the Doctors and all Medical Providers

Our Ailing Medical System

Sandeep Jauhar, M.D. authored and published *Our Ailing Medical System: American doctors are increasingly unhappy with their once-vaulted calling* (The Wall Street Journal, August 30, 2014), and *Doctored: The Disillusionment of an American Physician* (2014). In his insightful writings, Dr. Jauhar showcases the struggles of doctors in America, "We trained [doctors] with ideals and high standards, now to be clerks typing on keyboards and mouse clicking boxes." He goes on to say, "[a] majority of doctors express diminished enthusiasm for medicine and say they would discourage a friend or family member from entering the profession."

Over the years, there have been talks of doctors going on strike. We believe that they already have. Medical students have been striking for decades and chose not to enter certain specialties. As a result, we do not have enough primary care physicians to meet the needs of our population. Many physician extenders, like Physician Assistants (P.A.) and Nurse Practitioners (N.P.) are foregoing primary care to enter specialty fields. We do not contest the rights of practitioners to enter their preferred area of medicine. We do, however, believe that primary care has been overburdened to the point of being avoided as a practice option.

You Must Prove Everything You Do

Fours years ago, we received a notice from UVWX[56] insurance plan regarding the quality of care for our patients with Diabetes mellitus. The plan discovered 104 instances of poor care, meaning that we did not obtain A1c or LDL "bad" cholesterol blood tests or microalbumin urine tests during a given calendar year. The result of the report was to decrease our quality payment rewards and label us as a "poor quality" office.

The UVWX report confused us. We followed a protocol and were attentive to ordering the proper tests. In addition, we discussed the results of the tests with our patients, and used them to measure the severity of their diseases. We were puzzled. Why didn't the insurance company know that the tests were performed? After all, they paid for the tests! The company representative explained that patients often change their insurance plans; so, it is hard to track whether a patient underwent a test, paid for by their company. We did not believe the answer.

We invited our UVWX insurance company representative to meet with us, and we piled all 104 charts on our lunchroom table. One by one, we went through the paper charts. After reviewing each chart, we had zero deficiencies for A1c, LDL or urine microalbumin testing.

About 40 people on the list had not obtained their yearly dilated retinal diabetic eye examination. This test can only be done by an eye doctor (Ophthalmologist/Optometrist). The insurance company rules, however, stipulated that if the patient did not go to an eye doctor and get a yearly diabetic eye exam, then the primary care provider would be punished —as if no quality measures were achieved for that patient – for the entire calendar year.

The insurance company representative said that she understood our position and "agreed to disagree" on the plan's policy toward primary care physicians. She said it was "up to us doctors to figure out a solution."

---

56 "UVXY" is a factitious name used for this story.

Part of the solution: EHR's, Patients and Doctors/Providers

Part of the solution will come from using electronic health records (EHR's), part of it will come from doctors/providers, and the rest will come from all of us, as patients.

EHR's

Though EHR's have been disruptive to the practice of medicine, the benefits of quality analysis will eventually shine. Doctors will no longer be held hostage by potentially erroneous insurance company or government quality reports. EHR systems will gain the ability to seamlessly track quality measures. They will display results in table and graph forms and indicate when each task is due for completion. Patients, providers and insurance/government plans will have instant access to quality reports.

"The medical office of the future will have a patient, the doctor, a computer and a dog. The dog will be there to bite the doctor if he touches the computer."

This joke has been around for a long time in reference to aircraft pilots. In the pilot version, one could view it as an insult to pilots. We are not suggesting, however, that computers should replace pilots, and we do not question their expertise. Pilots use the computer as a tool and are not offended by the joke. An Apache combat pilot and instructor explained to us, "I often tell my students to let go and allow the computer to fly the craft." He acknowledged the advantages of technology, but adds, "There is something special about looking over a battlefield with human eyes." He also cited instances where emergency human pilot landings resulted in saved lives – while later computer simulations were all unsuccessful.

By analogy, medical practitioners sense the need to have engagement with patients in order to use the best of human intelligence. EHR's do have their place in healthcare. When it comes to tracking and monitoring purposes, the EHR is a master. We believe that the worst of EHR adoption is behind us, as most practices have converted from written to electronic records. Rather than waiting for an insurance company or government audit, EHR's will display a continual audit report. This will help medical providers and patients to work together to assure high quality, while tailoring action to the needs of individuals.

The Patient

Patients will exercise their rights to facilitate their healthcare. Laws support their ability to view their health record and request amendment to correct errors or inadequate information. Laws will emerge to allow patients to "remove from view" or archive other information. Medical providers have an opportunity to guide their patients on how to do this. We recommend that providers encourage their patients to view their health records before and after medical encounters. We recommend that patients keep an open mind regarding the use of a Pre-History and work with medical staff to accommodate their ability to co-author the history component of their health record.

> *Every right implies a responsibility:*
> *Every opportunity, an obligation,*
> *Every possession, a duty.*
> *John D. Rockefeller (1839-1937)*[57]

As patients gain confidence in their newfound advocacy rights, they will become powerful drivers of healthcare policy. With the transparency of health records, patients will be able to recognize bureaucratic red tape. Patient responsibility, obligation and duty will emerge to transform the practice of medicine. As physicians and medical providers, we must

---

57 Rockefeller, J.D. (n.d.). Retrieved December 27, 2014, from http://www.brainyquote.com/quotes/quotes/j/johndrock147463.html

take a leadership role in promoting the best interest of our patients while strengthening the patient-provider relationship.

Doctors/Medical Providers

Promoting the review of health records before and after each encounter will likely spawn a variety of responses from patients. Handling these patient responses and allowing patients to co-author their health records sounds like an avalanche of time-consuming, burdensome tasks. "Over eighty percent of physicians indicate that they are already overextended or are at full capacity."[58] How can we expect more? As physicians who have successfully run a private practice, we understand the concern of exceeding the limits of our capacity. We are protective against additional tasks that threaten to disrupt patient-provider engagement.

We know that when physicians are asked, "What two factors do you find MOST satisfying about medical practice?," physicians rank highest: patient relationships (78.6%) and intellectual stimulation (65.3%).[59] These responses override financial rewards (15.2%) and prestige of medicine (12.2%). As doctors, we want to engage with our patients and function at our highest level of education. Transferring written health records to a digital format has required physicians to function as clerks — in a manner that has disrupted the patient-provider relationship. Medical practices have felt and will continue to feel the growing pains of new technology. We see this coming to an end as EHR systems continue to interoperate, smoothly function and seamlessly track quality data. We expect a re-awakening of the practice of medicine as the patient-provider relationship morphs into a partnership.

According to HIPAA Privacy Rule CFR § 164.526, doctors have the right to refuse "a request for amendment," which means that you can

---

58 2014 Survey of America's Physicians, © Sept 2014, The Physicians Foundation
59 Ibid, p. 13, 18.

refuse a patient's pre-history. However, you are required to take action within sixty (60) days of the request.[60] We are *not* in favor of creating more paperwork. We recommend, therefore, that you allow your patients express themselves to their own levels of satisfaction, so as to "co-author" the History section of their health record with the consistent use of a pre-history.

Because newfound patient rights are based on federal law, patient participation is inevitable and imminent. We wrote this guidebook with attention to federal law and EHR/billing format so as to standardize the patient and the doctor/medical provider responses. These rules of engagement are intended to guide the application of law with an outlined approach to foster the patient-provider relationship. Allowing patients to exercise their federal rights might well be the best thing that has ever happened to your medical practice.

When we discuss the patient-provider partnership, we focus on a display of empathy. As previously reported, high physician empathy is associated with better clinical outcomes and greater patient satisfaction. Not surprisingly, it also results in greater physician satisfaction. We do not view patient empowerment as an impediment to physician duties but, rather, welcome new roles in which patients and doctors/providers work together.

In response to *Our Ailing Medical System*, five letters to the editor were published a week later in The Wall Street Journal. Four sympathized and affirmed the author's impressions. The fifth response, offered by a doctor, proposed "an even simpler cure for his medical malaise: Do your colleagues and patients a favor and retire already."[61] According to a 2012 survey, over 60% of physicians said they would retire today if they could.

---

60 HIPAA Regulations Section-By-Section Amendment of Protected Health Information: Right to Amend. (n.d.). Retrieved February 26, 2015, from http://www.bricker.com/services/resource-details. aspx?resourceid=386

61 "Do your colleagues and patients a favor and retire already" — letter to the editor, The Wall Street Journal, September 6, 2014.

This was up from 44.9% in 2008.[62] We sympathize and empathize with Dr. Jauhar. We do not feel that the solutions to our healthcare system should call for his retirement or the retirement of any of our medical practitioners. Rather, we propose physician/provider leadership in helping our patients participate in their care by effectively and knowledgeably utilizing modern technology to reduce burdens.

There's a Freight train Coming: ICD 10

Those thoughts of retirement may return as the United States updates from the International Classification of Disease (ICD) version 9 to version 10. Starting October 1, 2015, we will assign upgraded codes to all conditions and diseases. This sounds trivial until you try to do it. Think of the change as a freight train coming toward you, and you are on the tracks.

The World Health Organization (WHO) copyrights ICD for the purpose of having a worldwide coding system for the identification and organization of diseases and conditions. This is important because it unifies all scientists in the study of human health and disease. *Bertillon's International List of Causes of Death* is believed to be the first ICD in 1893.[63] Jacques Bertillon, M.D. was the Chief Statistician for the city of Paris. Dr. Bertillon's classification was adopted by many countries and eventually published by the Health Organization of the League of Nations. Over time, the World Heath Organization accepted responsibility for all subsequent revisions.

In 1977, the World Health Organization published the 9th revision of ICD. Since 1979, the U.S. has used the 9th edition with clinical modifications, as developed by the National Center for Health Statistics (NCHS), which is part of the U.S. Centers for Disease Control and Prevention (CDC). ICD-9-CM uses 13,000 codes to describe conditions, such as *sore throat (462)*, *finger pain (729.5)*, and *Diabetes mellitus, without mention of*

---

62 2012 Survey of America's Physicians, © Sept 2012, The Physicians Foundation, p. 83.
63 Principles & Practice of ICD-10 Coding, Verma, D., El-Sayed A.M., © 2009, p. 1A

complications type II or unspecified type, not stated as controlled (250.00). ICD-10-CM will use 70,000 codes when implemented on October 1, 2015 in the United States. Pain in the left finger (M79.645) will have a separate code from right finger pain (M79.644). ICD-10-CM requires more detail to choose the correct code. It demands greater specificity (what is wrong) and laterality (which side of the body).

Most countries of the world upgraded to ICD-10 in 1994. Our country has been kicking the can down the road for over two decades. An upgrade in 2005 would have been easier. After examining a patient and viewing an x-ray, a doctor could have written *initial encounter for a non-displaced fracture of the proximal phalanx of the left ring finger* and the medical coder would have assigned *S62.645A* ICD-10 code. Now, with the EHR, the doctor must figure out and enter the correct code into the computer before anything else can be done for the patient!

Take a 3-hour CME Approved Professional Coder Course Designed For Physicians

We recommend that all physicians/medical providers should be trained in ICD-10. The American Academy of Professional Coders (AAPC) has a course designed for you.[64] For less than $300, you can take a 3-hour online course, specifically designed for physicians. Doctors can choose among twenty-one specialties and gain three AMA PRA category 1 CME credits. We recommend doctors train now, so that they can get used to the detail and nuances of ICD-10. With this short course, doctors will be able to judge whether more training is necessary.

Some physicians argue that we should further delay upgrading from ICD-9-CM to ICD-10-CM. We cannot afford to wait any longer. We are trying to compare our healthcare quality, cost and satisfaction using

---

64 AAPC.com, ICD-10 Training for Physicians, 3 CME, $295, 800-626-2633 x4. As of January 18, 2015 and for a limited time, AAPC is offering a non-CME version of this course free for practices with fewer than 5 practitioners.

codes from the 1970's. Meanwhile, the rest of the world upgraded over two decades ago. We should not allow the ICD-10 freight train to disrupt and devastate our medical practices. We recommend that providers take a course, learn the lingo and get on the train.

Chapter 10

Expectations & Implementation

We wholeheartedly believe in patient advocacy rights and, to that end, we support the inevitable responsibilities, obligations and duties that will emerge for all stakeholders. We cite federal laws (PSDA 1990, HIPAA 1996, Privacy Rule as a final rule of HIPAA 2002) that are only now being realized. What sets our approach apart from other texts is our ability to implement practical solutions to healthcare. We theorize that our nation's lackluster scores for healthcare quality, cost and satisfaction can be improved by the rise of the patient advocate. To test our hypothesis, we have initiated a Patient Advocacy Initiative with Conemaugh-Duke Lifepoint Healthcare in Johnstown, Pennsylvania. With Internal Review Board (IRB) and Scientific Review Committee approval, we are implementing a study, *Patient, Provider and Medical Staff Experiences as a Measure of a Pre-History.*

We are preparing our providers and medical staff to recognize and accommodate patient advocacy rights described in this guidebook. We will monitor patient, provider and medical staff experience with surveys before and after pre-history use. We encourage patients to view their health record before and after all medical encounters, and promote shared decision-making while fostering a strong patient-provider relationship.

Because HIPAA does not have an age restriction, children patients also possess the rights and abilities outlined in this book. Beginning now, we are training a new generation. Therefore, we must be mindful of how we approach healthcare in the digital age.

You do not have to wait for us to conduct and publish research studies in order for you to be your own best advocate. While it will take some planning and accommodation by your medical provider to incorporate your pre-history into your electronic health record, you can immediately apply your newfound rights. If you seek care with a provider that has not been trained to be a patient advocate, we suggest that you bring a condensed version of a pre-history. You can describe only the Chief Complaint and History of Present Illness, if you like. As for the Status of your Chronic Diseases, do not hesitate to assemble information about your condition. Any and all medical facilities should be able to accommodate your few sentences by entering the content into the history part of your electronic health record.

The beauty of our patient advocacy approach is that there are no restrictions on age, gender, race, income status or geographic location with the U.S.

We must all pay close attention to the consequences of having *permanent* digital information. We will need to create mechanisms so to best track our health, but not infringe on our personal privacy.

We propose four recommendations for all of us as patients, doctors/providers, and the government.

For the doctors/medical providers:

1. Embrace electronic health records as a tool.
2. Encourage Patient Advocacy, which includes patient review of the health record before and after each encounter and the acceptance of a patient's pre-history.
3. Learn to use ICD-10.
4. Become involved in the process of regulating and protecting your patients' medical information.

For the Government:

1. Change the requirements for annual Wellness Exams and Annual Dilated Diabetic Retinal Examinations from once every twelve months to once every calendar year.
2. Expand CMS 1500 form field 21 from 4 to unlimited diagnostic codes. (at least support the NUCC in the expansion to 8 codes)
3. Stop using modifier 25 as a trigger to audit or bundle services.

4. Continue to enact legislation and utilize the best technology to secure and protect the medical information privacy of all citizens.

For all of us as Patients:

1. Review your health record with goals to understand your conditions while maintaining the accuracy and content of your medical story and, as needed, prepare for your medical encounter by composing a pre-history
2. Encourage the use of ONE patient portal that interoperates with all electronic health records.
3. Learn to manage your health and healthcare as a full-fledged partner with your doctor/medical provider.
4. Become involved with patient advocacy groups to assure that your voice is heard when institutions and governments create policies and laws regarding your health information.

Chapter 11

Conclusion

We started off by asking why anyone would want to look at their health records, and proceeded to describe newfound federal rights that have been enabled by electronic health records. We anticipated the consequences of having patients view their healthcare records and even explored the potential for patients to co-author a medical encounter. We have described a healthcare reformation, due to the rise of the patient advocate.

Because we are all patients of the healthcare system, patient advocacy affects all of us. As personal representatives, we can care for those we love with full support of the law.

Our country is in an unsteady state of transition when it comes to healthcare. We pay too much and get too little in return when it comes to quality and satisfaction. Our current pathway is financially unsustainable.

The missing piece of the equation is *you*. You have the ability and the right to greater participation in your healthcare. To a considerable degree, you have the ability to control your medical story for content and accuracy. This facilitates the potential to significantly improve your care, while reducing the cost. As a partner with your medical provider, you can choose among the best, most efficient, and cost-effective treatment options for you.

We expect patient and provider satisfaction to improve as we work together with a common set of expectations. With empathy, doctors/medical providers will be able to best understand your healthcare needs; and, with reciprocal empathy, you will understand the requirements that your providers face.

We anticipate costs to stabilize and reduce as fewer services and tests are duplicated. We also expect your accurate medical history to lead to more effective testing and treatment.

We expect quality measures to soar as you take an active role in managing your own healthcare.

"A new way of looking at something becomes successful only when the old way miserably fails."[65] Have we failed enough? Are we ready to ride the paradigm shift in healthcare? Are we ready for a Patient Advocacy revolution?

The patient advocacy revolution needs only use logic as its weapon. Let's welcome a new standard in medical care. Let's empower the client of healthcare to make crucial decisions. Let's respect personal representatives as an equal partner in patient care. Let's all work together.

Rise of the Patient Advocate was written because we believe that you, the patient advocate, are the driving force of our healthcare future. We want you to be satisfied with your healthcare. We also want you to consistently receive excellent care. We are convinced that it is possible to achieve high quality and high satisfaction while being cost-effective. We will conduct our research for more insight. Meanwhile, we invite you to be a patient advocate for yourself, with a view to controlling your healthcare outcome for your benefit and, ultimately, for society as a whole. It's all about doctors/providers who want to understand their patients, and patients who want to be heard.

We wish you a healthier and more enlightened future, and we invite you to discuss the issues raised in this text at greater length by visiting PatientAdvocacyInitiatives.org.

Yours in health and the healthcare partnership,

Drs. Michael & Margaret Warner

---

65 See tribute to Dr. Thomas Kuhn in Chapter 1.

About the Authors

Michael J. Warner, D.O., C.P.C. and Margaret K. Warner, D.O. have served the community of Ebensburg, Pennsylvania for over twenty years. They operated Warner Family Medicine, P.C. and are medical staff members of Duke LifePoint-Conemaugh Memorial Medical Center, Johnstown, PA. Drs. Warner are officers of Patient Advocacy Initiatives, a 501(c)(3) non-profit organization, registered in the state of Pennsylvania, with a mission to help patients become their own best advocates.

As physicians, patients, small business owners and employees, Drs. Warner have a unique perspective on healthcare. Dr. Michael Warner's certification as a professional coder adds additional insight into the practical functioning of the healthcare system.

Drs. Warner are both board certified in family medicine/osteopathic manipulative treatment by the American College of Osteopathic Family Physicians (ACOFP). Dr. Michael Warner is also board certified in neuromusculoskeletal medicine/osteopathic manipulative medicine by the American Osteopathic Board of Neuromusculoskeletal Medicine (AOBNMM). Drs. Warner are both graduates of Des Moines University – College of Osteopathic Medicine, Iowa. Dr. Margaret Warner has an undergraduate degree in biology from Michigan State University while Dr. Michael Warner has undergraduate degrees in biology and philosophy from Villanova University.

Both Drs. Warner are adjunct assistant clinical professors of family medicine at Lake Erie College of Osteopathic Medicine (LECOM).

The authors encourage you to learn more about Patient Advocacy at PatientAdocacyInitiatives.org and on Facebook.

Index

A

B

C

Criminal Activity 86

D

E

F

G

government 23, 25, 35, 40, 41, 42, 43, 50, 52, 85, 86, 87, 92, 93, 100
Guardian 31

H

handwritten 10, 23
health records 10, 11, 13, 14, 15, 20, 23, 24, 25, 29, 44, 45, 48, 49, 50, 76, 81, 82, 83, 84, 85, 87,
       88, 93, 94, 99, 102
healthcare 9, 10, 11, 12, 13, 14, 15, 16, 17, 18, 19, 20, 21, 22, 23, 25, 26, 28, 29, 30, 31, 32, 33,
       34, 35, 37, 38, 43, 44, 48, 49, 50, 51, 52, 53, 55, 63, 64, 65, 67, 68, 71, 73, 74, 75, 76, 82,
       84, 87, 92, 93, 95, 97, 99, 101, 102, 103, 105
healthcare system 17, 18, 20, 31, 34, 35, 37, 50, 95, 102, 105
Health Information Technology for Economic and Clinical Health Act (HITECH) 51
Health Insurance Portability and Accountability Act (HIPAA) 22, 23, 24, 77, 81, 82, 88, 99
History of Present Illness 57, 58, 61, 62, 63, 67, 69, 99
Human Curiosity 24
hysterectomy 24

I

Identifying and Implementing Quality Measures 25
immunization 26, 27
Implications of Refusing Treatment 27
Inaccurate Information 79
Incomplete Quality Measures and Patient Penalties 26
Increased Efficiency and Evidence Based Medicine 36
infant mortality rates 16
influenza 25, 27, 28, 36
Insufficient Documentation 78
interactive 20, 54
Interoperability 50

J

Jefferson Scale of Empathy 74

K

knowledge 18, 19, 24, 44, 46, 47, 53, 69, 77, 85

L

lab 10, 45, 85
Latin 18, 19, 24, 45, 56
law 22, 23, 24, 28, 29, 46, 76, 83, 95, 102
life expectancy 16

M

N

O

P